Instructor's Manual to Accompany Essentials of Diagnostic Microbiology

Lisa Anne Shimeld

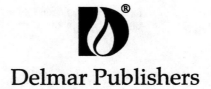

Delmar Publishers

an International Thomson Publishing company I(T)P

Albany • Bonn • Boston • Cincinnati • Detroit • London • Madrid
Melbourne • Mexico City • New York • Pacific Grove • Paris • San Francisco
Singapore • Tokyo • Toronto • Washington

NOTICE TO THE READER

COPYRIGHT © 1999
By Delmar Publishers
a division of International Thomson Publishing Inc.

The ITP logo is a trademark under license.

Printed in the United States of America

For more information, contact:

Delmar Publishers
3 Columbia Circle, Box 15015
Albany, New York 12212-5015

International Thomson Publishing Europe
Berkshire House
168-173 High Holborn
London, WC1V7AA
United Kingdom

Nelson ITP, Australia
102 Dodds Street
South Melbourne
Victoria 3205, Australia

Nelson Canada
1120 Birchmount Road
Scarborough, Ontario
M1K 5G4, Canada

International Thomson Publishing France
Tour Maine-Montparnasse
33 Avenue du Maine
75755 Paris Cedex 15, France

International Thomson Editores
Seneca 53
Colonia Polanco
11560 Mexico D. F. Mexico

International Thomson Publishing GmbH
Königswinterer Strasβe 418
53227 Bonn
Germany

International Thomson Publishing Asia
60 Albert Street
#15-01 Albert Complex
Singapore 189969

International Thomson Publishing Japan
Hirakawa-cho Kyowa Building, 3F
2-2-1 Hirakawa-cho, Chiyoda-ku,
Tokyo 102, Japan

ITE Spain/Paraninfo
Calle Magallanes, 25
28015-Madrid, España

JOIN US ON THE WEB: www.DelmarAlliedHealth.com

Your Information Resource!
- What's New from Delmar • Health Science News Headlines
- Web Links to Many Related Sites
- Instructor Forum/Teaching Tips • Give Us Your Feedback
- Online Companions™
- Complete Allied Health Catalog • Software/Media Demos
- And much more!

1 2 3 4 5 6 7 8 9 10 XXX 03 02 01 00 99 98

Library of Congress Card No.: 98-17226

ISBN 0-8273-7389-9

Contents

Introduction

Essentials of Diagnostic Microbiology is a new text that presents the essential, entry-level skills and information medical laboratory technology students will need to enter the workforce. The text encourages students to use their critical thinking skills to explore topics further, seeking additional information when necessary. Compared to other texts, this approach saves students and educators valuable time they would otherwise spend extracting essential information from the volume of material.

This Instructor's Manual is a companion to *Essentials of Diagnostic Microbiology*. It includes answers to the Review Questions found in chapters 1–51 of the student text, as well as suggested answers to the Case Studies contained in most chapters.

In addition to this Instructor's Manual, the following ancillaries are also available:

- *Study Guide and Laboratory Manual to Accompany Essentials of Diagnostic Microbiology* reinforces concepts presented in the text through numerous multiple choice, matching, short answer, labeling, and critical thinking questions corresponding to each of the text chapters. The second half of this study guide serves as a laboratory manual and contains step-by-step instructions on how to perform over fifty of the most common procedures done in a microbiology lab.

- *Computerized Testbank to Accompany Essentials of Diagnostic Microbiology* includes over 1,500 test true/false, multiple choice, labeling, and short answer test questions based on the contents of the text chapters.

Text Organization

Essentials of Diagnostic Microbiology contains fifty-one chapters that focus on the fundamental principles and techniques involved in the study of microorganisms, as well as their application in the diagnosis of infectious disease. A unique feature of this text is its emphasis on *essential* information presented in short, easy-to-understand segments. Five sections further subdivide the material into manageable parts. Each of the four subspecialty areas, Sections 2–5, include short introductory chapters that lay the groundwork of basic technical, biological, and chemical principles related to that specialty. Subsequent chapters within each section then build upon this information by describing the characteristics of microorganisms recovered in the clinical laboratory and the practical approach to their identification. The chapters cover the collection and processing of clinical specimens and the interpretation of laboratory investigative results, tracing the application of basic principles of microbiology and characteristics of microorganisms to the recovery and identification of infectious agents in the clinical laboratory. This organization from simple to complex allows students to build knowledge and confidence gradually, applying what they learn to the identification of microorganisms and the diagnosis of infectious diseases.

Section I, General Topics in Microbiology provides students with a concise overview of diagnostic microbiology. Chapter 1 introduces the learner to the study of microorganisms, while Chapters 2–7 focus on key topics such as the infectious disease process, laboratory safety, immunologic and molecular techniques, quality assurance, automation, and antimicrobial agents and antimicrobial susceptibility testing.

Section II, Bacteriology contains two parts: *General Methods for Identification of Bacteria and Isolation* and *Identification of Bacteria from Clinical Specimens*. Part 1 begins with an introductory chapter (Chapter 8) to ground learners in the basics of microscopic morphology, methods, techniques, and identification. Chapters 9–23 introduce students to the identification of the most common bacteria they may encounter in the clinical microbiology lab. Part 2 begins with a similar introductory chapter (Chapter 24) to introduce students to techniques in processing and interpreting cultures from clinical specimens. Chapters 25–33 take a body-systems approach to introduce the common resident flora of that system, specimen collection, specimen processing, related pathogenic microorganisms, and diseases.

Section III, Mycology begins with two introductory chapters (Chapters 34 & 35) that present the basic concepts and techniques related to mycology, including a review of fungi, approaches to identifying fungi, and media techniques, specimen collection and transport, and direct examination of specimens. Chapters 36–41 cover superficial and subcutaneous mycoses and dimorphic, opportunistic, and saprobic fungi and yeasts.

Section IV, Parasitology also begins with an introductory chapter (Chapter 42) that reviews basic concepts and techniques related to parasitology, including symbiotic relationships, hosts, disease transmission, life cycles, and an overview of important parasites.

Chapters 43–47 next cover specimen collection and processing, protozoans, and helminths.

Section V, Virology covers basic virology concepts, including specimen collection and processing, and concludes with a special chapter on emerging viral infections.

The text also includes a comprehensive glossary comprising all the key terms listed in each chapter.

Key Features

The unique learning aids included in *Essentials of Diagnostic Microbiology* are detailed in the **Key Features** section on pages xiv–xv of the text. Often, students are unfamiliar with the value of such learning aids. I suggested walking your students through this two-page spread to familiarize them with the text and point out the usefulness of these learning aids. These features include:

Microbes in the News — Real-life news stories about microbiology "in action" provide interesting chapter lead-ins and foster classroom discussion. You may also ask students to find news items on the Internet or in medical journals or ask them to follow up on the items presented in the chapters to see if anything has changed.

Outline — A list of the main topics and subtopics previews each chapter's major points. Encourage students to review these topic headings *before* beginning a chapter. Also remind students that the outlines will serve as good study guides for tests, in conjunction with the learning objectives.

Key Terms — Unfamiliar or critical vocabulary words are listed alphabetically at the beginning of each chapter and appear in boldface when first used. These terms are later defined in the Glossary. Encourage students to make flashcards of the key terms to test themselves or each other.

Learning Objectives — The objectives identify the key information to be gained from the chapter. Remind students that after studying a chapter they should review the learning objectives to ensure they have mastered each one.

Procedures — Abbreviated instructions on how to perform specific laboratory procedures appear throughout the text. Each one includes an overview of the procedure, principle, method, quality control, expected results, and references. The student text has a complete list. All of the text procedures, plus many others, are included in more detail in *Study Guide and Laboratory Manual to Accompany Essentials of Diagnostic Microbiology*.

Color Plates — The text includes an insert of color plates with detailed captions of many of the organisms discussed within the chapters. The plates are numbered consecutively and referenced within the text for easy use. See the beginning of the text for a complete index of color plates.

Summary — Each chapter summary is presented in a bulleted format, emphasizing the key points from the chapter, to help students focus their study.

Case Study — Case studies provide a critical thinking scenario for students to put their knowledge of content into practice.

Review Questions — Multiple choice questions at the end of each chapter challenge students on the material they have just learned for quick reinforcement of concepts. The answers appear in the *Instructor's Manual*.

References & Recommended Reading — This listing includes both the references used in each chapter, plus additional sources for further study.

CHAPTER 1

Introduction to the Study of Microorganisms

Answers to

Review Questions

1. Gram-positive cells are purple after decolorization because:
   - **d. they retain the crystal violet through decolorization.**

2. The term "coenocytic" refers to:
   - **a. fungal hyphae that lack septa between nuclei.**

3. In the classification of life kingdoms represent _____ taxonomic group.
   - **b. the largest and least specific**

4. A pellicle is:
   - **d. a flexible covering found on some protozoans.**

5. A microbiologist examines a preparation of cells. Even when magnified 1000X the cells are tiny, with no apparent nucleus or organelles. The majority of these cells are arranged in chains. What kind of cells are they?
   - **d. Streptococci**

6. The dramatic decline in leprosy cases that occurred between 1985 and 1994 can be primarily attributed to:
   - **c. the implementation multidrug therapy introduced by WHO.**

7. Chitin is:
   - **b. a lipid that causes *mycobacterium* to stain acid fast.**

8. Plasmids are:
   - **d. small, circular DNA molecules found in some bacteria.**

9. Which of the following is found in most procaryotic cells but is never found in eucaryotic cells?
   - **d. Peptidoglycan**

10. Endospores are produced by:
    - **c. six genera of gram-positive bacteria.**

11. "Bacterial species" is a difficult concept to define. Which of the following contributes to the problem?
    - **a. It is not possible (or relevant) to evaluate reproductive compatibility between bacteria because they usually reproduce asexually by binary fission.**

12. A protozoan is detected in a blood specimen. The organisms are elongated, leaf-shaped, and possess a flagellum. The organism is a member of which phylum and subphylum?
    - **b. Sarcomastigophora, mastigophora**

13. Multicellular organisms with flattened bodies divided into segments are likely to have which of the other following characteristics?
    - **b. No digestive system**

14. Which of the following is a characteristic of fungi but not plants?
    - **d. All of the above**

15. The identity of isolates of a clinical sample is determined by:
    - **c. comparing the characteristics of the isolate to those of known organisms until a match is achieved.**

16. Members of the same class are also members of the same _____.
    - **d. Phylum**

17. Which of the following are criteria used to classify fungi into phyla?
    - **c. Type of sexual spore produced**

18. Specialized organ systems will be present in:
    - **c. helminths.**

19. Tapeworms possess:
    - **b. segmented bodies.**

20. Which of the following is NOT one of the five kingdoms proposed by Whittaker?
    - **b. Viridae**

CHAPTER 2

The Infectious Disease Process

Suggested Answers to

CASE STUDY 1: VARIATION IN HOST SUSCEPTIBILITY TO *Listeria*

From January to August 1985, a county hospital in Los Angeles documented 142 cases of symptomatic listeriosis. The source of the bacteria was a certain brand of Mexican-style soft goat cheese. Ninety-three of the infected individuals were fetuses or newborns; the other 49 were adults (75% were pregnant women). Thirty infants and 18 adults died as a result of the infection. Forty-eight of the 49 infected adults were immunosuppressed (due to pregnancy, drugs, or illness) or elderly.

Many female goats and sheep harbor *Listeria monocytogenes* in their genital tracts and mammary glands. These hardy bacteria can grow at refrigerator temperatures and can survive within phagocytic leukocytes. The cheese plant followed safety regulations during the pasteurization process of the milk. The problem appeared to be that the flow of milk through the pasteurization equipment was too fast. Consequently, some raw milk got into the final product. (Adapted from Schuchat, A., et al. [1991]. Epidemiology of human listeriosis. *Clin Microbiol Rev.*, 4:169–183.)

Questions:

1. Propose possible changes in the processing procedures that could reduce or eliminate the risk of future contamination problems with *L. monocytogenes*. **Set up a quality control procedure to monitor the flow of milk through the equipment.**

2. Why did this disease affect only pregnant women, infants, and fetuses? **Because they were either immunocompromised or did not yet have a functional immune system. The pregnant woman was immunocompromised due to being pregnant. In a manner of speaking, her fetus could be considered an antigen. Infants do not have fully functional immune systems for the first couple of years of life and therefore are more susceptible than the general population. The fetus does not yet have a functional immune system.**

3. Explain why a microbiologist might place a portion of a food specimen at 4°C for 5 to 7 days, before subculturing onto selective media for *Listeria*. **To allow the bacteria to grow under what are really selective conditions (lowered temperatures) before plating.**

Answers to

Review Questions

1. Which of the following mechanisms is NOT part of the host's innate resistance?
   c. **Secretion of immunoglobulins by plasma cells**

2. Endotoxin is:
   d. **a toxic lipid that is a component of the outer membrane of gram-negative bacteria.**

3. *Cryptococcus neoformans* avoids phagocytosis by:
   a. **producing a large polysaccharide capsule.**

Suggested Answers to

CASE STUDY 2: BACTERIAL ENDOPHTHALMITIS CAUSED BY A SOIL BACTERIUM, *AGROBACTERIUM RADIOBACTER*.

The pathogenicity of an organism is related to the site of infection as well as the immune status of the host. A 70-year-old man underwent uneventful outpatient cataract surgery with sutures. Four days later, he returned to the eye clinic with orbital swelling, a purulent discharge, and pain in the sutured eye. He did not have a fever. He did report that he had worked in his garden on the evening of his discharge.

Vitreous fluid was aspirated and submitted for Gram stain and culture (aerobic and anaerobic). The Gram stain showed a moderate number of short pleomorphic gram-negative rods with leukocytes. No growth was seen on the anaerobic cultures, but a heavy, pure growth of nonhemolytic colonies was seen on the sheep's blood agar as well as the MacConkey's plates (incubated aerobically). The Vitek GNI card identified the bacteria as *Agrobacterium tumefaciens (A. radiobacter)*; 98% probability. The patient was given empirical therapy: steroids to reduce inflammation and a combination of vancomycin and gentamicin. He recovered completely.

Human infections with Agrobacterium are rare. They are soil organisms and those that contain the Ti plasmid produce crown gall disease or hairy root disease in plants. Although the two species are indistinguishable biochemically, human isolates are referred to as *A. radiobacter*. (Excerpts from case study by Miller, Novy, & Hiott [1996]. *J Clin Microbiol* [1996]. 34:3212–3213.)

Questions:

1. Discuss the factors involved in the development of this rare bacterial infection. **The surgery and suturing of the eye allowed for entry of the bacterium. The patient must have unconsciously rubbed his eye, introducing the soil-dwelling bacterium.**

2. Why did the lab set up anaerobic as well as aerobic cultures on the vitreous fluid? **The interior of the eye is an anaerobic environ- ment. Also, many soil dwellers are anaer- obes, and the patient had reported working in his garden.**

3. Discuss the pros and cons of outpatient surgeries. **Pros include lowered costs, possi- bly less chance of nosocomial infections. Cons include the lack of trained supervision to monitor patient progress/condition.**

4. The ability of a microbe to cause disease depends on the host's:
   d. **all of the above**

5. When microbial antigens mimic host tissue they may:
   d. **all of the above**

6. Superantigens are:
   c. **unusual exotoxins that bind nonspecifi- cally to receptors on helper T lympho- cytes and cause overproduction of IL-2.**

7. *Helicobacter pylori* can survive in the stomach because they:
   d. **produce urease and form ammonia.**

8. *Mycobacterium tuberculosis* avoid killing by the cells of the immune system by:
   b. **surviving within phagocytic white blood cells.**

9. Phase variation:
   b. **involves the switching "on or off" of genes for various characteristics.**

10. *Treponema pallidum* slow the activation of acquired immunity by:
   a. **coating themselves with albumin**

CHAPTER 3
Safety in the Clinical Microbiology Laboratory

Suggested Answers to

CASE STUDY

A microbiologist, wearing contact lenses, failed to protect his eyes with safety glasses and had a speck of preserved fecal specimen enter his eye. He removed his contact lens, washed out the affected eye, and replaced the lens. Several hours later his eye became irritated. He again removed his contact lens and washed his eye, but this time he did not replace the lens. By the following day, his eye became very painful and he reported to Employee Health. He was quickly hospitalized with a critical eye injury.

The doctor reported that the severity of the injury may have been greatly lessened if the technologist had obtained medical assistance promptly instead of trying to treat himself and if the contact lens had not been replaced after the first washing.

Questions

1. The technologist was working with a preserved fecal specimen. What safety items should he have been using? **Gloves, goggles or face shield, gown, or other protective items that would have helped him avoid physical injury.**

2. Knowing the nature of the specimen what two types of injury would you suspect when his eye became irritated? **Two possible types of injury are chemical injury from the preservative and infection from the organisms in the feces.**

3. The doctor in Employee Health made some suggestions about the eye injury. What other suggestions would you make? **Other suggestions are: a. Make sure that an ophthalmologist is called in on consult for the hospitalized technologist. b. Put the accident information in the employee's file. c. Hold an employee inservice training about the PPE and the first aid procedures for spills and splashes in the laboratory.**

Answers to

Review Questions

1. When investigating infections, the route of transmission would be of prime importance. The most common routes of transmission in the laboratory are:
   d. **oral, respiratory, percutaneous, and cutaneous.**

2. As indicated by the focus of regulations, the greatest potential risks for laboratorians are associated with the:
   b. **processing of primary clinical specimens.**

3. The CDC-NIH has issued guidelines and OSHA has issued the *Standard*. The microbiologist should know that the:
   c. ***Standard* is a federal regulation requiring mandatory compliance.**

4. Encouraging laboratory workers to use safety equipment and personal protective equipment (PPE) is an important part of good laboratory practices. The most effective way to promote this use is:
   b. **education sessions on the devices.**

5. All health care institutions should have a written policy for:
   b. **spills of blood and body fluids.**

6. The Centers for Disease Control and Prevention (CDC) has published lists of organisms and classified them in biologic safety levels (BSLs). Two organisms of concern, human immunodeficiency virus (HIV) and *Mycobacterium tuberculosis* (TB), would be dealt with at the greater security of BSL:

   c. 3

7. "Sharps" is a category covering needles, scalpel blades, fragile glass, and pipets. Needles are not to be recapped or bent before disposal. To avoid transmission of HBV or HIV, all sharps are to be placed in:

   a. red molded plastic boxes.

8. Standard Precautions include the use of gloves when appropriate:
   1. for blood and body fluids.
   2. with nonintact skin.
   3. when answering a laboratory phone.
   4. for opening laboratory doors.
   5. while training in new procedures.

   b. 1, 2, 5

9. Infectious droplets carrying tubercle bacilli are easily passed from a coughing patient or accidental breakage of liquid suspensions of TB. Consequently the infection rate with TB among clinical and laboratory personnel is almost eight times higher than the general population. Good safety practices when dealing with potential TB situations involve:
   1. educating and skin testing of employees.
   2. use of respirators when working.
   3. vaccination of new employees.
   4. proper directional airflow in the laboratory.

   a. 1, 2, 3, 4

10. When cleaning a spilled culture in the laboratory, one should wear a gown and gloves. To decontaminate the spill area which solution would be best to use?

    b. 1:10 dilution of sodium hypochlorite

CHAPTER 4
Immunologic and Molecular Techniques

Answers to

Review Questions

1. B lymphocytes have a life span:
   b. of one to two weeks.

2. The role of IgG in the immune system is:
   d. a and b are roles of IgG.

3. Phagocytic cells in tissues are known as:
   d. macrophages.

4. When stained with Wright's stain which of the following contain coarse red granules?
   c. Eosinophils

5. When stained with Wright's stain which of the following contain coarse blue-black granules?
   b. Basophils

6. B cells recognize and bind specific antigens with:
   a. receptors on their surface.

7. The test that results in lines of identity, partial identity, or non-identity is the:
   b. Ouchterlony test.

8. The polysaccharide capsule of *Streptococcus pneumoniae* inhibits:
   a. phagocytosis by macrophages.

9. IgA:
   d. is secreted in mucous membranes.

10. IgE:
    a. is produced in response to some parasitic infections.

CHAPTER 5

Quality Assurance in the Clinical Microbiology Laboratory

Answers to

Review Questions

1. Collection personnel need instructions on:
   d. **all of the above.**

2. Assessment of the quality of a specimen can be made by:
   b. **monitoring the span of time from collection to time of receipt.**

3. The quality of reagents is maintained by:
   d. **a and c**

4. Quality control of instruments:
   b. **is dictated by the manufacturer.**

5. A properly labeled specimen:
   c. **has date and time of collection.**

6. Trends are:
   d. **data published for physicians to examine how treatment regimens are affecting the patient.**

7. Procedure manuals are of value because:
   d. **all of the above**

8. Procedure manuals must have which of the following?
   b. **a and c**

9. If results of quality control tests are outside the expected values:
   c. **the test must be repeated before reporting results**

CHAPTER 6

Automation in the Clinical Microbiology Laboratory

Answers to

Review Questions

1. An automated test assay that uses antibody labeled with horseradish peroxidase:
   d. **could be detected via a color change if the labeled antibody reacts with the proper substrate.**

2. Radioimmunoassay (RIA):
   b. **has largely been replaced by ELISA.**

3. Gas-liquid chromatography (GLC):
   a. **may be used to rapidly identify mycolic acids of mycobacteria.**

4. Automated mycobacterial identification systems:
   c. **usually must rely on specimen decontamination and concentration before inoculation of media.**

5. Which of the following is NOT a characteristic of blood culture systems?
   b. **Blood culture systems can directly identify microorganisms from the blood culture bottle without the need for subculturing.**

6. Automated methods:
   d. **tend to save technician time in the clinical microbiology laboratory.**

7. PCR/LCR:
   a. **may be used to identify microorganisms directly from clinical samples.**

8. Turbidometric methods:
   c. **may be used in automation to measure antibiotic susceptibilities.**

9. Some automated enzyme immunoassay systems are designed to detect antigens from:
   a. ***Chlamydia trachomatis.***

10. Instruments that identify microorganisms (such as Aladin, Microscan, Vitek, etc.):
    d. **often may identify gram-positive, gram-negative, and anaerobic bacteria, and yeast.**

CHAPTER 7

Antimicrobial Agents and Antimicrobial Susceptibility Testing

Answers to

Review Questions

1. Microbistatic substances help combat microbial infections by:
   c. **attacking something that the microbe requires.**

2. Which of the following affects the administration of antimicrobial drugs given to humans?
   d. **All of the above**

3. It is more difficult to attack microbial cell membranes because:
   b. **of the similarities to human cell membranes.**

4. Drugs like the polymyxins are used primarily as:
   b. **topical agents.**

5. Toxicity in the administration of the aminoglycosides is due primarily to:
   d. **their buildup in the patient's system.**

6. The tetracyclines:
   c. **effectively penetrate the body.**

7. Macrodilution broth sensitivity tests of antimicrobial agents are:
   b. **too expensive and time consuming to use routinely.**

8. The Kirby-Bauer method is:
   a. **a standard disk diffusion method used to establish the effectiveness of antimicrobial drugs.**

9. Which of the following affect the choice of chemotherapeutic agents in the treatment of infectious disease?
   d. **All of the above**

10. The polyenes:
    d. **Both a and b are true.**

CHAPTER 8

Microscopic, Cultural, and Other Techniques for Bacterial Identification

Suggested Answers to

CASE STUDY

The microbiology technician who was reading plates at the urine culture bench encountered the following:

The blood agar plate that was to be used for a colony count was found to have a single line of very heavy growth down the center of the plate. This growth was such that colonies were indistinguishable although bacterial swarming was present surrounding the apparent line of inoculation. The remainder of the plates were streaked using the three-quadrant method.

Considering the standard method for streaking a urine culture and bacterial characteristics, in general, answer the following questions:

Questions:

1. Was an error made streaking the plate for colony count? If so, what was it and can the plate be used for its intended purpose? **The plate for colony count was streaked incorrectly. The initial streak was made down the center (presumably with a calibrated loop), but the cross streaks at 90° angles were not made. All of the bacteria are growing along the line of inoculation. The plate cannot be used to determine a colony count, since colonies are not distinguishable.**

2. What would be the next step for completing the work on this culture? **If the remaining plates appear to be a pure culture and are not contaminated with skin flora, identification of the causative bacteria should be made and reported.**

3. How should the results of this culture be reported? Why? **The bacterial identification and antibiotic sensitivities should be reported to the physician. However, it is not possible to do a plate count to include in that report. The omission of this material should be reported according to departmental policy.**

4. What may have caused the swarming of the bacteria? **Bacterial swarming is a characteristic of certain very motile bacteria and may give a hint to the technician regarding the identification of the bacteria.**

Answers to

Review Questions

1. The media that is NOT differential is:
   c. **nutrient agar.**

2. A slide preparation to test for motility is a:
   d. **wet mount.**

3. A mordant:
   b. **makes stain more intense.**

4. In a Gram stain, the safranin serves as the:
   d. **counterstain.**

5. *Mycobacterium tuberculosis* is suspected. A direct smear of the sputum is prepared. The correct way to stain this smear is with:
   d. **Ziehl-Nielsen stain.**

6. The bacitracin disk is used to inhibit the growth of:
   a. *Streptococcus* **group A.**

7. Streaking a urine culture uses:
   b. **a calibrated loop.**

8. Reducing media is used for cultivation of:
   c. **anaerobic bacteria.**

9. Complete hemolysis of the area surrounding a colony is known as:
   b. **ß-hemolysis.**

10. A colony that appears to be yellow and is coagulase positive most likely is:
    c. *Staphylococcus aureus.*

11. Anaerobic culture techniques require the use of a system where the oxygen has been removed or utilized. When using a system of this type, the colorless strip in the jar indicates that the:
    a. **oxygen has been removed.**

12. A candle jar contains conditions of:
    b. **reduced oxygen.**

13. The reagent used to perform the catalase test is:
    b. **hydrogen peroxide.**

14. When performing a Gram stain, round, purple bacteria and long, pink bacteria are seen. This smear should be read as having:
    b. **gram-positive cocci and gram-negative rods.**

15. A known culture of micrococcus is Gram stained. It appears to be pink, cocci. These results are:
    c. **incorrect because the bacteria should appear gram-positive.**

CHAPTER 9

Staphylococcus and Related Aerobic Gram-Positive Cocci

Suggested Answers to

CASE STUDY 1: OSTEOMYELITIS AND SEPTIC ARTHRITIS

An 11-year old boy was admitted to the hospital because of spiking fevers. He also complained of right knee pain, and although there had been no known injury, he was active in football and enjoyed in-line skating. His mother had been giving him acetaminophen for the low-grade fever and pain for about a week.

On admission, he developed severe pain and tenderness in the right leg and a fever of 39.4°C. Radiographs were negative. Aspiration of the knee produced fluid with 3,500 leukocytes/mm³ with 86% neutrophils. A bone scan was "hot" in the distal tibia of the right leg. Bacterial cultures were ordered on blood, joint fluid, and a tibial aspirate. The next day, cream-colored colonies surrounded by a large zone of ß-hemolysis were seen on blood agar plate from all sites. Gram stain of the isolates revealed gram-positive cocci, in pairs and clusters.

Questions:

1. What colonial and cellular morphologic features indicate a staphylococcal infection? How would you differentiate streptococci from staphylococci? **ß-Hemolytic colonies are typical of *S. aureus*. Gram-positive cocci in pairs and clusters, as opposed to chains, would indicate a staphylococcal isolate. Staphylococci divide in multiple planes, whereas streptococcus divide in single planes, tending to form chains, especially when grown in a liquid medium or stained from clinical material. The catalase test is the primary test used to differentiate staphylococci (catalase-positive) from streptococci (catalase-negative).**

2. This patient has septic arthritis (infected joint) and osteomyelitis (bone infection) with *S. aureus*. What test would then be performed to identify this isolate as a *S. aureus*? What activities may have increased this boy's risk for infections of this type? **Trauma that may have occurred from football or skating can infrequently lead to these infections. Portals of** entry can include superficial wound infection (which may be inapparent), or hematologic spread from another infected site.

3. What other type(s) of infections can this organism cause? **See Table 9–2, Diseases Associated with *S. aureus*.**

4. What types of antimicrobial resistance can this organism exhibit? What are the mechanisms of resistance? How is resistance detected in the clinical microbiology laboratory? ***S. aureus* can be resistant to many antimicrobics, including ß-lactamase-resistant penicillins and cephalosporins. *S. aureus* produces ß-lactamases and can also alter penicillin-binding proteins that lead to frank methicillin resistance. Heterogeneous populations of methicillin resistance can be missed if careful adherence to NCCLS standards is not followed. Special considerations include an incubation temperature that does not exceed 35°C, a full 24-hour incubation of disk diffusion tests, and using salt-supplemented media (as with oxacillin screen agar).**

Suggested Answers to

CASE STUDY 2: CATHETER-RELATED SEPSIS

A 42-year-old man had a history of leukemia that required a bone marrow transplant 6 months ago. He experienced numerous hospitalizations and required a long-term central venous catheter (right subclavian port-a-cath) for ongoing medication.

The patient had been in the hospital for a scheduled follow-up for 7 days the previous week. Four days after hospitalization, he developed fever, chills, and pain at his central line insertion site. He drove himself to the hospital where his temperature was recorded at 38.5°C. Physical examination revealed right upper extremity swelling.

Aerobic and anaerobic blood cultures were drawn into commercial vials of broth media (one set through the port-a-cath and one set via a peripheral vein), and placed into an automated blood culture instrument. Both sets of blood cultures were positive at 24 hours for gram positive cocci. The positive cultures were subcultured to nonselective media to identify the organisms.

Questions:

1. What is the most likely cause of this infection? Why did the positive vials have to be subcultured prior to identification? What tests will be used to identify this organism? **The increased use of long-term indwelling devices, such as port-a-caths, has caused an increase in CNS-related sepsis. Blood cultures are in broth media, and Gram stain alone cannot establish identity. Therefore blood cultures must be subcultured to a solid medium for traditional identification procedures to be performed. Once grown, catalase and coagulase tests would be used to identify organisms as CNS, the majority of which are *S. epidermidis*. Other commonly recovered CNS include *S. hominis*, *S. haemolyticus*, *S. warneri*, *S. simulans*, and *S. cohnii*. However, complete speciation using reference methods is labor-intensive and time-consuming. Kits and automated methods are limited in their ability to accurately identify unusual CNS, so clinical laboratories rarely speciate isolates.**

2. How could one determine that these isolates were the same organism? **A similar biotype or antibiograms might indicate identity, although this is not very sensitive. Increased availability and standardization of molecular methods such as PFGE will facilitate these determinations. However, these techniques should be reserved to prove identity of strains in problematic cases or nosocomial infection investigation.**

3. Why is it significant that both sets of blood cultures were positive? **A single blood culture drawn from one site may represent organisms picked up during venipuncture (skin contamination), whereas drawing two cultures from separate sites is a considerably better indicator of infection.**

4. Vascular access catheters are frequently removed if they appear to be infected. How are catheters handled (for culture) in the microbiology laboratory? **CNS are adherent because of physical interactions (e.g., hydrobonding, hydrophobic interaction) between the cell wall and indwelling devices. Some strains produce an extracellular polysaccharide "slime" layer, which makes these organisms more adherent and protects them from host defenses.**

Suggested Answers to

CASE STUDY 3: MRSA IDENTIFICATION

A 74-year-old diabetic woman was taken to the emergency room from her nursing home because of hip pain and fever. She had a long history of infected foot ulcers, which were typically treated with antimicrobics, surgical debridement, or both. Admission temperature was 101°F, and her white blood cell count was elevated at 18,000 mm³, with a predominance of neutrophils. Magnetic resonance imaging of the pelvis indicated a possible access in the inguinal area. Blood cultures and aspirates were positive with an organism with the following characteristics:

Medium-sized, nonhemolytic white colonies grew on blood and chocolate agars, with no growth on MacConkey agar. Gram stain showed gram-positive cocci in pairs and clusters. The isolate was catalase positive and negative with a commercial latex agglutination test used to differentiate *S. aureus* from the CNS. The technologist recorded a preliminary report as CNS with antimicrobic susceptibilities to follow. On the following day, susceptibilities by disk diffusion showed multiple resistance, including a heteroresistant pattern around the oxacillin disk. The technologist remembered that this patient had previously been identified as having been colonized with MRSA in axillary and groin cultures, and performed additional tests to confirm her suspicion that this was actually an MRSA isolate.

Questions:

1. What additional tests could be performed to prove that this was an MRSA? **This isolate may not have reacted with the latex product because of an alteration in the expression of protein A (clumping factor), by being masked by a capsule, or by an actual reduction of these cell wall–bound coagulase. Additional tests which could be used to identify this isolate include the tube coagulase and second generation latex kits.**

2. What suggested that this might be an MRSA? **Although CNS can be resistant to multiple antimicrobics, the heteroresistant pattern around the oxacillin disk and the patient's history of colonization increased the suspicion that this might not be CNS.**

3. What was unusual about the colonial morphology (i.e., not typical of an MRSA isolate)? **Most *S. aureus* will be ß-hemolytic and will be easily identified by catalase and most latex products. There has been some difficulty with misidentified MRSA using the latex products. This has been addressed by some manufacturers by incorporating antibodies to MRSA capsular antigens into their product.**

4. What test would then be performed to identify this isolate as *S. aureus*? **MRSA are nosocomial agents, which tend to be found in tertiary care facilities, teaching hospitals, and long-term facilities, such as nursing homes. They are transmitted by patient-to-patient contact with hospital personnel who are not using proper handwashing techniques or by patients coming in contact with items from another MRSA patient. Factors favoring colonization include prior antibiotic use and periodic hospitalization in facilities that house MRSA.**

Answers to

Review Questions

1. What Gram stain morphology does *S. aureus* have?

   b.   gram-positive cocci in clusters

2. What Gram stain morphology do *Micrococcus* species have?

   b.   gram-positive cocci in tetrads

3. The following might be used to identify *S. epidermidis* except:

   d.   ß-lactamase reaction.

4. A blood culture from an intravenous drug abuser grows out a gram-positive coccus with the following characteristics: catalase positive, coagulase negative, multiply drug resistant. What is the most likely organism?

   a.   *Staphylococcus epidermidis*

5. A young woman is seen for symptoms of a urinary tract infection. Although her urine culture only grows out 20,000 cfu/mL, it is in pure culture. The technologist uses the following tests to identify the isolate: catalase positive, coagulase negative, novobiocin resistant, naladixic acid resistant, nitrofurantoin susceptible. The organism is:

   d.   *S. saprophyticus.*

6. Staphylococcal food poisoning is characterized by:

   c.   a 2 day–2 week incubation period.

7. *S. epidermidis* is associated with all of the following except:

   d.   toxic shock syndrome.

8. A positive blood culture shows gram-positive cocci in tetrads. The following day yellow pigmentated colonies are observed. Catalase and modified oxidase reactions are both positive. What is the most likely organism?

   c.   *Micrococcus* species

9. Detection of *mec*A in staphylococcal isolates would be useful in determining what type of antimicrobial resistance?

   a.   oxacillin

10. A wound culture grows out gram-positive cocci with the following characteristics: ß-hemolytic colonies that are both catalase and coagulase positive. What is the most likely organism?

    b.   *S. aureus*

CHAPTER 10

Streptococcus and Related Aerobic Gram-Positive Cocci

Suggested Answers to

CASE STUDY 1

A 51-year-old woman presented with fever and shaking chills for 4 days. She was febrile and had marked tenderness over the right rib cage. A chest radiograph showed lesions indicative of septic pulmonary emboli. Abdominal computed tomography showed involvement of hepatic parenchyma and hepatic veins. *Streptococcus anginosus* was isolated from culture of a hepatic aspirate from the lesion and from blood cultures. *S. anginosus* is part of the normal flora of the skin and mucous membranes. Portal of entry to the patient's bloodstream was not apparent.

Questions:

1. Discuss how to identify to the species level viridans streptococci isolated from blood cultures. **By using commercial biochemical tests, such as the RaPID STR system.**

2. Why is it important to definitively identify viridans streptococci isolated from blood cultures? **Because they may be associated with infective endocarditis in patients with damaged native valves. They may also be isolated from specimens of neutropenic patients.**

CASE STUDY 2

A previously healthy 29-year-old man presented with high fever, swelling, and marked tenderness of the left thigh. Ultrasonography showed a hypoechoic area between the subcutaneous and muscle tissue. A clinical diagnosis of necrotizing fasciitis was suspected. Early treatment with antibiotics was indicated. A deep incision to the fascia was performed. After verification of the diagnosis, radical debridement of all necrotic tissue resolved the focus. Necrotizing fasciitis is caused by an invasive strain of *Streptococcus pyogenes*. The initial process involves inflammation and occlusion of muscle vessels followed by fascia necrosis. The necrosis spreads to subcutaneous tissue so that the swelling is observed before cutaneous signs appear. Early treatment with antimicrobics and surgical intervention are critical to preserve the patient's limb and life.

Questions:

1. The invasive strain of *S. pyogenes* that cause necrotizing fasciitis may cause a higher rate of more serious infection in children and in the elderly compared to the rest of the population. Explain. **Children and the elderly are somewhat immunocompromised. Children do not have fully developed immune systems, and in the elderly, the immune system is declining.**

2. A swab from infected tissue was sent to the laboratory for culture. What plating media should one choose to ensure the isolation of ß-streptococci? **Stab into sheep blood agar so that if streptolysin O is produced it can be detected.**

Answers to

Review Questions

1. This microorganism is the most virulent species in the genus *Streptococcus* and is responsible for suppurative sequelae such as rheumatic fever and glomerulonephritis.
   b. *S. pyogenes*

2. Choose the most likely organism with the following characteristics and clinical significance: gram-positive cocci implicated in pneumonia of newborns and puerperal fever in postpartum females; ß-hemolytic on sheep blood agar, CAMP factor positive, hippurate hydrolysis positive.
   c. *S. agalactiae*

3. A gram-positive coccus that is strongly associated with dental caries and belongs to a heterogeneous group of streptococci best characterizes this species.
   a. *S. mutans*

4. This group of organisms forms tiny colonies on blood agar, satellite around colonies of staphylococci and can cause endocarditis.
   c. *S. defectivus*

5. Emerging multiply resistant strains of this organism are becoming a major problem in the hospital environment. This bacterium grows in 6.5% NaCl and hydrolyzes esculin in the presence of bile salts.
   d. *E. faecalis*

6. This virulence factor acts by preventing opsonophagocytosis. It is localized in the fibrils, which are attached to the peptidoglycan of streptococcal cell wall.
   a.   M protein

7. Isolation of this organism from blood cultures of a patient is indicative of a possible bowel malignancy. It is bile esculin positive but does not grow in 6.5% NaCl.
   c. *S. bovis*

8. A common cause of community-acquired pneumonia, these pathogens may appear as α-hemolytic mucoid colonies or small colonies with a crater-like center. They are optichin positive and are highly autolytic.
   b. *S. pneumoniae*

9. Necrotizing fasciitis is an invasive infection of muscle and fat tissues. Mortality is high unless the disease is rapidly diagnosed, the wound is surgically debrided, and antibiotic therapy instituted. The etiologic agent is:
   d.   group A streptococcus.

10. A compromised host is:
    b.   more susceptible than other individuals to opportunistic infections.

CHAPTER 11

Aerobic Gram-Positive Bacilli, Coccobacilli, and Coryneform Bacilli

Answers to

Review Questions

1. What organism is not often encountered in the average hospital except in areas where industries related to cattle are found ?
   d. *Bacillus anthracis*

2. An acute communicable disease, characterized by upper respiratory tract infection, and systemic toxin effects, caused by the Klebs-Loeffler bacillus is:
   c. diphtheria.

3. This organism resembles *Nocardia* and *Actinomyces,* an opportunistic pathogen found in the human oral cavity, which can cause abscesses and endocarditis.
   c. *Streptococcus pyogenes*

4. The localized cellulitis often on the hand, arm, or fingers of animal and animal product processors, caused by *Erysipelothrix rhusiopathiae* is:
   c. erysipeloid.

5. Primarily a disease of cattle, sheep, goat, and horses, which disease caused by a *Bacillus* species can be contracted by humans working with these animals?
   b. Anthrax

6. The *Bacillus* species that often causes food poisoning due to nondestruction of its spores by normal cooking temperatures is:
   a. *Bacillus cereus.*

7. A form of anthrax characterized by a malignant pustule is:
   c. cutaneous anthrax.

8. A food-borne reportable disease linked to many epidemics since 1981, caused by *Listeria monocytogenes,* is
   b. listeriosis.

9. Frequently found in the Gram stain or culture of a healthy vagina, playing a protective role from gonococcal infection and bacterial vaginosis, which organism is occasionally involved in human infections?
   b. *Lactobacillus acidophilus*

10. The term used to denote a club-shaped bacillus or an irregularly shaped gram-positive rod is:
    a. coryneform.

CHAPTER 12
Aerobic Actinomycetes

Suggested Answers to

A 20-year-old Mexican-American woman presented to the surgical clinic with a lump in the right popliteal fossa. She reportedly had had two resections of the lesion over a 6-year period in Mexico. Nevertheless, it continued to manifest intermittent drainage. She also complained that it became painful on exposure to cold or after prolonged standing. She had no history of trauma and a questionable history of knee injury. Physical examination revealed two scarred circumscribed subcutaneous nontender nodules, each approximately 0.5 cm in diameter, and about 3 cm apart, in the right popliteal fossa. No drainage was noted, and no masses or cysts were palpated.

Two apparent sinus tracts and a contiguous scarred area in the subcutaneous tissue of the popliteal fossa were explored. Two small nodules were noted in the mass, one of which was sectioned, revealing brown fluid, which was submitted for routine culture only. The remaining specimen was sent for pathologic examination. (Braunstein, Hicks, & Konyn, 1990)

Questions:

1. Given the patient's history, what diagnoses should be considered? **Clinical symptoms suggest actinomycetoma. *Nocardia brasiliensis* is the causative agent for skin and subcutaneous infection as a result of a skin puncture induced by plant material. *Nocardia* can be differentiated from *Streptomyces* and *Actinomadura* by the modified Kinyoun stain. *Nocardia* species are partially acid-fast, whereas *Streptomyces* and *Actinomadura* are not.**

2. What qualities, growth characteristics, and biochemical studies will be required to identify the organism once it is isolated? **Nocardia brasiliensis is a slow grower. The biochemical reactions would include hydrolysis of casein, tyrosine urea, and esculin. The organism fails to hydrolyze xanthine.**

3. How is the therapeutic approach influenced by the nature of the organism? **Nocardia will respond to sulfonamide therapy but not to penicillin. Modified Kinyoun prep must be performed to differentiate aerobic from anaerobic *Actinomycetes* agents.**

Answers to

Review Questions

1. Which one of the following organisms are partially acid-fast when stained with the modified Kinyoun stain?
   d. none of the above

2. The key to differentiate *Nocardia brasiliensis* from other *Nocardia* species is the hydrolysis of casein, tyrosine, and:
   a. failure to hydrolyze xanthine.

3. A kidney transplant patient developed a temperature and cough. Pulmonary x-ray showed pulmonary infiltrate. Gram-positive branching rods were observed on the Gram stain. Modified Kinyoun stain was performed. The rods were partially acid-fast. The organism grew aerobically. The etiologic agent is probably:
   c. *Nocardia* species.

4. The most commonly encountered pathogenic aerobic actinomycete from clinical samples is:
   c. *Nocardia* species.

5. Aerobic actinomycetes:

    d. **all of the above**

6. The key biochemical to differentiate *Nocardia* species from *Actinomadura* species is:

    a. **lyzozyme broth.**

7. Which aerobic actinomycete is the causative agent for maduramycosis?

    d. **none of the above**

8. Which aerobic actinomycete is the causative agent for pulmonary, systemic, and cutaneous diseases, including mycetomas?

    d. ***Nocardia* species**

9. The causative agents for localized infections involving bone, cutaneous, and subcutaneous tissue are:

    a. ***Nocardia, Streptomyces, Actinomadura.***

10. The second most commonly encountered pathogenic aerobic actinomycete from clinical samples is:

    b. ***Actinomadura* species.**

CHAPTER 13

Neisseria and Other Aerobic Gram-Negative Cocci

Suggested Answers to

CASE STUDY

A previously healthy 3-month-old infant girl was seen in the Emergency Department for fever and lethargy. Her temperature was 40.5°C (105°F). She had a 1-day history of vomiting and irritability. She was noted to have muscle rigidity, a pulse of 130, respiratory rate of 45, and blood pressure 165/65. A lumbar puncture was performed and revealed purulent material showing numerous leukocytes, predominantly neutrophils on Gram stain. Bacteria were seen both intracellularly and extracellularly. CSF protein was 1200 mg/dL; the glucose level was 8 mg/dL. Several hours later the child developed a diffuse, petechial rash. Blood cultures were drawn and grew the same microorganism as was isolated from the CSF.

Questions:

1. What is the likely diagnosis for this patient's infection? What is the infectious agent? How do you know? **The diagnosis is meningitis with meningococcemia. The infectious agent is *Neisseria meningitidis*. This bacterium appears morphologically as gram-negative diplococci. A petechial rash caused by bleeding and coagulopathies frequently accompanies infection.**

2. Explain the need for prompt examination of a gram-stained smear to rapidly diagnose this infection. **Fulminant meningococcemia may**

be rapidly fatal. Rapid deterioration may be accompanied by development of shock, disseminated coagulopathy, and organ failure. The key to successful treatment is early recognition of disease and prompt institution of appropriate antibiotic therapy.

3. What recommendations would you make to protect members of the patient's immediate family from developing this infection? **Close contacts of patients with meningococcemia must receive immediate prophylaxis with appropriate antibiotics to prevent disease.**

Answers to

Review Questions

1. The member of the genus *Neisseria* that is always considered to be pathogenic is:
   b. *N. gonorrhoeae.*

2. Which test is positive for all *Neisseriae* and *Branhamella catarrhalis?*
   c. **Oxidase test**

3. Which statement is correct?
   d. **Gonorrhea is spread by direct contact.**

4. *Branhamella catarrhalis* is a:
   a. **gram-negative coccus.**

5. Selective media for the isolation of *N. gonorrhoeae* include:
   d. **all of the above**

6. *N. gonorrhoeae* is capnophilic; this means that it:
   c. requires a high concentration of CO_2.

7. An enzyme that can hydrolyze antibiotics such as penicillin is:
   c. ß-lactamase.

8. *Branhamella catarrhalis* is apt to cause which type of infection?
   b. Pneumonia

9. A particularly fulminant disease associated with the meningococcus is called:
   c. Waterhouse-Friderichsen syndrome.

10. The following species of *Neisseria* is (are) able to produce a starchlike polysaccharide from sucrose:
   d. *N. mucosa.*

CHAPTER 14
Haemophilus

Suggested Answers to

CASE 1: INFANT WITH MENINGITIS DUE TO *H. INFLUENZAE* TYPE B

An 8-month-old boy was brought to the emergency room by his parents because the child had suddenly become irritable and was experiencing breathing difficulty. While in the emergency room the child vomited and had a convulsion. The physician noted that the patient had a stiff neck and a fever of 39.8°C. A lumbar puncture was performed and blood was collected for culture. Laboratory analyses revealed a cloudy cerebrospinal fluid (CSF) with 25,400 white blood cells/mm³ (97% were neutrophils), an elevated level of protein of 1,421 mg/dL (normal range is approximately 15–45 mg/dL) and a low glucose concentration of 19 mg/dL (normal is approximately 40–80 mg/dL). Numerous white blood cells and small gram-negative coccobacilli were found in stained smears of the CSF (thus ruling out *S. pneumoniae* as the causative agent). A latex agglutination test performed on the sample was positive for the type b capsular polysaccharide of *H. influenzae*. Culture of the CSF on chocolate agar showed the typical colonial growth of *Haemophilus*. Blood cultures were also positive. A diagnosis of meningitis due to *H. influenzae* type b was made. The infant responded well to intravenous infusions of ceftriaxone and was discharged from the hospital the following week.

Questions:

1. Are the given signs and symptoms specific for meningitis due to *H. influenzae* type b? **There are no signs or symptoms that specifically identify *H. influenzae* type b as the causative agent in a pediatric case of meningitis. Examples of other bacteria that may result in a similar clinical presentation include *Streptococcus pneumoniae* and *Neisseria meningitidis*. Young children with this syndrome are often treated with antibiotics that are effective against all three of these organisms.**

2. What other types of specimens could have been tested? **A urine sample is often tested by the latex agglutination technique, using specific bacterial antigens. Patients with meningitis may present with a rash—i.e., purpuric or petechial skin lesions. In these cases, fluid from a lesion may be Gram-stained and cultured.**

3. Is there a vaccine that could have prevented the disease? **Several vaccines consisting of purified type b polysaccharide that is attached to a protein, such as the outer membrane protein of *N. meningitidis* and diphtheria toxoid, are approved for use. These conjugated vaccines are T lymphocyte–dependent, inducing a greater antibody response against the type b polysaccharide than the original nonconjugated version. Since these newer vaccines are highly effective and immunizations are given early in life (2, 4, and 6 months of age), it is likely that this case of meningitis could have been prevented.**

Suggested Answers to

CASE 2: CHANCROID IN A PROMISCUOUS DRUG ADDICT

A 28-year-old man recently returned from the Mardi Gras in New Orleans presented with ulcerative lesions on the genitalia. The ulcers were soft and painful. On questioning the patient admitted to crack cocaine addiction and prostitution in exchange for the drug. Gram stains of exudate from the lesions showed pleomorphic gram-negative rods arranged in groups and chains. Most of the organisms were intracellular. No growth was evident on IsaVitaleX-supplemented chocolate agar until after 6 days of incubation in air containing 10% CO_2. A diagnosis of chancroid due to *H. ducreyi* was made and the patient was treated successfully with erythromycin.

Questions:

1. Did the promiscuous nature of the patient increase his risk of acquiring chancroid? **Since chancroid is a sexually transmitted disease, the more sexual partners one has, the greater is the risk of becoming infected with *H. ducreyi*. Promiscuity and ulcerative lesions are also associated with a number of other infectious agents, including *Treponema pallidum* (syphilis), *Calymmatobacterium granulomatis* (granuloma inguinale or donovanosis), and herpes simplex virus type 2 (genital herpes).**

2. How can *H. ducreyi* be differentiated from *H. influenzae*? **H. influenzae requires both hemin (factor X) and nicotine adenine dinucleotide (NAD, or factor V), whereas H. ducreyi requires only the V factor.**

Mueller-Hinton–based chocolate agar containing both factors and vancomycin is a standard medium for isolating both species. *H. ducreyi*, however, is a more fastidious organism, and its growth on the medium is slower. In addition, *H. influenzae* is positive for the catalase enzyme, whereas *H. ducreyi* is negative.

3. Is erythromycin the best antibiotic to use for *H. ducreyi*? **Erythromycin, ceftriaxone, and trimethoprim sulfamethoxazole are among the three most commonly used antibiotics for chancroid. However, treatment failures have been reported with the latter two. Essentially, all isolates of H. ducreyi are susceptible to erythromycin.**

Answers to

Review Questions

1. Which of the following statements apply to *Haemophilus?*
   a. **They are facultative anaerobes.**

2. Chocolate agar is used for the isolation of *Haemophilus* species because it provides the organisms with:
   b. **heme and nicotinamide adenine dinucleotide.**

3. The primary virulence factor associated with *H. influenzae* is:
   d. **a polyribose ribitol phosphate capsule.**

4. A small gram-negative coccobacillus isolated from a patient with conjunctivitis is MOST LIKELY to be:
   d. **H. influenzae biogroup aegyptius.**

5. The most common bacteria causing meningitis in young children aged 6 months to 3 years is:
   a. **H. influenzae type b.**

6. Identify the correct statement regarding the new conjugated vaccines for *H. influenzae*.
   d. **They induce protection against H. influenzae infection for up to 3.5 years.**

7. Which of the following is a sexually transmitted species of *Haemophilus* that causes chancroid?
   c. **H. ducreyi**

8. Identify the correct statement regarding the characteristics of *Haemophilus* species.
   b. **Haemophilus satellites around colonies of Staphylococcus aureus because the staphylococci secrete V factor.**

CHAPTER 15

Miscellaneous Fastidious Aerobic and Facultative Gram-Negative Bacilli and Coccobacilli

Suggested Answers to

CASE STUDY 1

A 23-year-old man is seen in the emergency room for an infected wound on his hand. The wound is swollen, feverish, and red, and a moderate amount of pus has accumulated at the site. On questioning, the patient explains that he was involved in a fist fight at a local night club 1 week earlier. During the fight, he had hit the other man involved in the mouth and broken several of his teeth, at which time he was bitten deeply by his opponent. The wound is a result of that bite. The physician lances the wound and bacterial culture of the drainage is performed.

After 48 hours incubation in 10% CO_2, tiny opaque colonies with a pale yellow pigment are observed on blood agar and chocolate agar plates. The organism Gram stains as a small gram-negative bacilli. Colonies are oxidase positive and catalase negative.

Questions:

1. What organism is the most likely pathogen isolated in this example? What was the source of the organism? **Eikenella corrodens is normal flora in the human mouth and likely was inoculated into the hand from the bite incurred during the fight.**

2. What other common colony characteristics would be helpful in presumptively identifying this organism? **Eikenella corrodens often "pits" the agar and emits a distinct bleach-like odor.**

CASE STUDY 2

A specimen on a 3-year-old girl is received from a pediatrician's office labeled "leg wound drainage." At 48 hours, small grayish nonhemolytic colonies are observed on blood and chocolate agars. Although the colonies Gram stain as gram-negative bacilli, there is no growth on MacConkey agar. A distinct "musty" or "mushroom-like" odor is detected, and the colonies demonstrate a positive oxidase result.

Questions:

1. Based on the information given, what organism do you suspect? What further background information would you request from the pediatrician's office to support your suspicions? **Pasteurella multocida is normal flora in the mouths of dogs and cats and is therefore a frequent pathogen in animal bites. The specific nature of the "leg wound" would be helpful. Is it a dog or cat bite?**

2. The cause of the "musty" odor can be determined by a spot bench test useful in identifying this organism. What test should be performed to assist in identification? **Pasteurella multocida demonstrates a strongly positive spot indole test; the indole is the cause of the odor.**

3. The suspected organism can be screened for based on sensitivity to a common antibiotic. What is the screening procedure often used? **Kirby-Bauer, because of its sensitivity to penicillin.**

Suggested Answers to

CASE STUDY 3

A 37-year-old man was admitted to a local hospital complaining of a severe headache of several days, moderate fever, chest pain, and a productive cough. Swollen lymph nodes and a tender, enlarged liver were also noted. He is a professional furrier and trapper and had recently returned from an excursion on which he had trapped and skinned approximately 30 rabbits.

Routine sputum and blood cultures were collected and inoculated aerobically and anaerobically onto routine media (blood agar plate, MacConkey agar, and CA, MAC). Although Gram stains of both the blood and sputum seemed to demonstrate the presence of very faintly staining gram-negative coccobacilli, no growth was obtained on any of the cultures after 72 hours.

After 6 days, the chocolate agar plates from the blood culture began to grow tiny transparent colonies of the organism. These colonies were oxidase negative and weakly catalase positive. Unable to conclusively identify the organism using any of their routine methods, the laboratory sent the isolate to a reference laboratory.

While awaiting the final identification results from the reference laboratory, the patient's pneumonia condition worsened, complicated by liver failure, and he died 3 weeks following admission.

Questions:

1. Given the patient's history and symptoms, what disease and organism do you suspect has infected the patient? *Francisella tularensis,* **most commonly contracted through direct or indirect contact with wild animals, causes tularemia.**

2. Assuming the laboratory was aware of the patient's specific history, describe the special precautions that should have been taken when working on specimens from this patient. **Working with suspected *Francisella* requires Biosafety Level 3 precautions.**

3. Why did the organism only grow on chocolate agar? Name two other types of media on which the organism will grow well. *Francisella* **species require cystine to grow. This is provided from Isovitalex. Cystine-glucose-blood agar and buffered charcoal yeast extract agar will grow *Francisella* species easily.**

Answers to

Review Questions

1. Of the following gram-negative organisms, which are commonly capable of growing on MacConkey agar?
   d.   none of the above

2. A suspected isolate of *Pasteurella* can be identified by its susceptibility to:
   c.   penicillin.

3. A patient develops a nonspecific disease several weeks following receiving a gift of Mexican goat cheese. A gram-negative coccobacilli is isolated from the patient's blood cultures. Based on this information, what is the most likely organism present?
   c.   *Brucella*

4. Even though *Gardnerella vaginalis* causes postpartum and neonatal bacteremia and septicemia, it will not be identified in blood cultures using most common systems because:
   d.   growth of *Gardnerella* is inhibited by the sodium polyanethol sulfonate present in many blood culture collection medias.

5. *Legionella* was probably not recognized prior to 1977 because:
   d.   both a and b are true.

6. Which bacterial media is best for isolation of *Legionella* species?
   b. **Buffered charcoal yeast extract agar**

7. A drug addict with visible "tracks" on his arm develops an infection among the lesions. The organism isolated is a tiny gram-negative bacilli that grows on blood agar but not MacConkey, is oxidase positive, and a majority of the colonies "pit" the agar. What is the most likely pathogen?
   a. *Eikenella corrodens*

8. It is common practice for dentists to prescribe prophylactic penicillin 2 weeks prior to any dental work on patients with a history of any heart defects to avert possible endocarditis. This would most likely be to prevent infection with:
   c. *Cardiobacterium hominis*

9. Which of the following are likely to result in contraction of tularemia?
   a. **Trapping and skinning of wild rabbits**

10. Which of the following would constitute the BEST diagnosis of "bacterial vaginosis"?
    b. **Observation of "clue cells" in a milky white vaginal discharge emitting a "fishy" odor**

CHAPTER 16
Gram-Negative Enteric Bacilli

Suggested Answers to

CASE STUDY 1: SEVERE DIARRHEA DUE TO ENTEROHEMORRHAGIC *E. COLI*

A previously healthy 9-year-old boy was awakened by excruciating abdominal cramps, nausea, and copious watery diarrhea every 30 to 60 minutes. He was brought to the emergency room later that evening when it appeared that there was bright red blood in his stool. Because of the severe nature of the illness, he was admitted to the hospital. The boy had no known contact with other persons with diarrhea and no history of recent travel outside of the United States. Symptoms appeared 24 hours after eating a hamburger at the local fast-food restaurant. It was determined that the patient had an elevated white blood cell count, but no fever. Erythrocytes, but no leukocytes, were found in the stool. Edema, erythema, and exudation were observed in the wall of the ascending and transverse colon during sigmoidoscopy; ulcers and pseudomembranes were not noted. There was concern that the infection may progress to hemolytic uremic syndrome, but urine tests were repeatedly normal. Routine cultures of stool revealed no *Salmonella*, *Shigella*, *Yersinia*, or *Campylobacter* and microscopic examination for enteric ova and parasites were negative. A sorbitol-nonfermenting *E. coli*, believed to be of the O157:H7 serotype, was recovered from the stool. The serotype was later confirmed by the State Public Health Laboratory. Antibiotics and intravenous fluids were administered over the next few days. The boy's stool was negative for the *E. coli* isolate by the time he was discharged from the hospital.

Questions:

1. Is the consumption of hamburger significant in this case history? **In the early 1980s, public health officials became acutely aware that severe hemorrhagic enteritis and hemolytic uremic syndrome could occur after consumption of undercooked hamburger. The meat was found to be contaminated with *E. coli* serotype O157:H7. Since then, this serotype has been associated with multiple food-borne outbreaks, and a variety of foods have been implicated. Contaminated ground beef, however, remains the most common source of the organisms. Healthy cattle appear to be a major reservoir for the organisms; meat becomes contaminated with intestinal contents from the animals during slaughter and processing.**

2. Why does this serotype of *E. coli* produce such severe illness? **The pathogenesis of serotype O157:H7 and other enterohemorrhagic *E. coli* (EHEC) is poorly understood. One toxin that the organisms produce is virtually identical to the bacteriophage-encoded verotoxin of *Shigella dysenteriae*. The severe nature of the infection thus may be related, at least partly, to direct effects of the toxin on epithelium and endothelial cells of blood vessels. Attaching and effacing proteins encoded by the *eae* gene and a strong inflammatory response against the bacteria are also likely to contribute to tissue destruction.**

3. Can *E. coli* O157:H7 be identified by means other than serotyping? ***E. coli* O157:H7 can be differentiated from most other *E. coli* in that it does not use sorbitol, is negative in the MUG test, and forms black colonies on certain types of commercially available agar. Serotyping of *E. coli* is performed primarily by reference laboratories. Other enterohemorrhagic *E. coli* include serotypes O26:H11 and some O111 isolates. Testing for specific virulence factors can also be performed by certain reference and research laboratories.**

Suggested Answers to

CASE STUDY 2: *KLEBSIELLA PNEUMONIAE* IN A CHRONIC ALCOHOLIC

A 55-year-old male transient stumbled into the emergency room of a large county medical facility. He was pale, coughing, and complaining of chest pain. "Rales," indicative of alveolar involvement, were heard on auscultation. Physical examination revealed an underweight, undernourished man with a rapid respiratory rate of 38/min, a temperature of 102.3°F, and alcohol on his breath. On questioning he admitted to "sipping" a pint of gin a day. Chest x-ray showed extensive consolidation with cavity formation in the lower right lobe of the lung. A bloody sputum was obtained by tracheal suction because the patient had difficulty in providing a specimen on his own. Numerous encapsulated gram-negative rods and a large number of neutrophils were noted. Cultures of the sputum for *Streptococcus pneumoniae*, *Mycoplasma pneumoniae*, and *Legionella pneumoniae* were negative; a heavy growth of *Klebsiella pneumoniae* was obtained. Despite high doses of broad-spectrum antibiotics, the patient's condition worsened and he was provided with a mechanical ventilator. The patient died of septicemia shortly thereafter.

Questions:

1. Why did antibiotic therapy in this patient fail? **K. pneumoniae can cause severe pulmonary disease, even in nonelderly subjects, if they have certain predisposing conditions, such as chronic alcoholism. Pneumonia due to these organisms is relatively common in alcoholics. In addition, the case history does not give the specific antibiotics that were used. Many isolates are now resistant to commonly used broad-spectrum antibiotics. Extended-spectrum second- and third-generation cephalosporins may have been more effective.**

2. Do other *Klebsiella* species cause respiratory tract disease? **K. ozaena and K. rhinosclero-** **matis, both of which are rare in the United States, can affect the upper respiratory tract. K. ozaena causes a progressive atrophy of the nasal mucosa, whereas K. rhinoscleromatis is the cause of a destructive granuloma of the nose and pharynx.**

3. Can *K. pneumoniae* be rapidly differentiated from other members of the *Enterobacteriaceae* family? **A presumptive identification of K. pneumoniae can be rapidly made if the organism is a nonmotile, lactose-fermenting, gram-negative rod with an unusually large, gelatinous capsule.**

Answers to

Review Questions

1. A midstream "clean-catch" urine from an asymptomatic 30-year-old pregnant woman yields numerous motile, lactose-positive organisms that are susceptible to common antibiotics. Which organism is MOST LIKELY responsible for the infection?

   b. *Escherichia coli*

2. Which of the following is a nonmotile organism with a large gelatinous capsule that can be found in the respiratory tract, as well as the intestinal tract, of healthy humans?

   c. *Klebsiella*

3. A picnic feast of potato salad, chicken, and hamburgers was consumed during a family reunion on a hot summer day. Within 24 hours eight family members experienced diarrhea, fever, and abdominal pain, which lasted for 2 days. Three people were eventually hospitalized and H_2S-producing gram-negative bacilli were isolated from the stool. Which of the following is the MOST LIKELY organism?

   d. *Salmonella typhimurium*

4. Microscopic examination of the stool from a patient with diarrhea revealed numerous red and white blood cells and mucus. A nonmotile, gram-negative rod that failed to ferment lactose was isolated from the stool. Blood cultures were negative. Which of the following is MOST LIKELY to be the causative organism?

   d. ***Shigella sonnei***

5. A gold miner in the southwest who develops the symptoms of bubonic plague is determined to have had contact with a/an:

   a. **rodent.**

6. Identify the MAJOR factor in *Yersinia pestis* that is associated with virulence, as well as the induction of protective immunity.

   d. **Fraction I**

7. Which of the following organisms is MOST LIKELY to cause a watery diarrhea?

   b. **Enteropathogenic *E. coli***

8. A common nosocomial pathogen with "swarming" motility is:

   c. ***Proteus mirabilis.***

CHAPTER 17

Nonfermenting Aerobic Gram-Negative Bacilli

Suggested Answers to

CASE STUDY 1: *PSEUDOMONAS AERUGINOSA* INFECTION IN A PATIENT WITH LEUKEMIA

A 15-year-old girl with acute lymphocytic leukemia went into remission while in the hospital. She was discharged, but was continued on long-term maintenance chemotherapy for the disease as an outpatient. Within 2 weeks she developed a slight fever and mild respiratory distress, but no other symptoms. However, her condition worsened rapidly and she returned to the hospital. At arrival her pulse rate and breathing were rapid and her temperature was 102°F. Laboratory analyses revealed that her white blood cell count was 0.3×10^9/L (significantly below normal). A combination of tobramycin and ceftazidime was initiated. Within hours, however, the patient's breathing became more labored, requiring intubation and respiratory assistance with a mechanical ventilator. Hypotension and shock due to low blood pressure were circumvented by the intravenous administration of fluids and drugs. Blood specimens taken during the first 2 days of hospitalization were positive for *P. aeruginosa*. Subsequent samples were negative. The patient improved slowly over the next few days and was eventually discharged. Chemotherapy for the leukemia was discontinued until her white blood cell count was above 1.0×10^9/L.

Questions:

1. Does leukemia predispose to developing *P. aeruginosa* infection? **Leukemia consists of progressive proliferation of abnormal leukocytes that are present in hematopoietic organs and other tissues. Since these cells are major components of the immune system and often do not function properly in patients with leukemia, there is increased risk for infection with a variety of agents. Chemotherapeutic drugs that are administered to patients with leukemia can also be immunosuppressive. Neutropenia is considered to be the major risk factor for infection with aerobic gram-negative bacteria, such as *P. aeruginosa*, although *E. coli* is the most commonly identified cause of bacteremia or sepsis in these individuals. Infection with *P. aeruginosa* becomes a significant concern when the absolute neutrophil count falls below 500/mm^3. Trimethoprim sulfamethoxazole is often given to patients with leukemia to prevent bacterial infections and pneumonia due to *Pneumocystis carinii*.**

2. What are the mechanisms by which *P. aeruginosa* enters the blood circulation? **Bacteremia following localized infection of burns or wounds with *P. aeruginosa* is a common and frequently fatal consequence. The organism produces numerous factors that contribute to its virulence, including elastases that destroy the walls of blood vessels and degrade the extracellular matrix of connective tissue. It appears that exotoxin A may also promote invasion into the blood circulation by inhibiting protein synthesis.**

3. What types of laboratory tests were likely to be used to identify *P. aeruginosa* in the blood specimens? **The organisms in the blood specimens were probably first isolated on blood agar and differential media. Characteristics that would help identify the isolates as *P. aeruginosa* include a large zone of ß-hemolysis around colonies growing on the blood agar, emission of an odor resembling that of overripe grapes, production of pigment (especially pyocyanin and pyoverdin), ability to grow on selective media such as EMB and McConkey's agar, and inability to ferment lactose, glucose, and other sugars.**

Suggested Answers to

CASE STUDY 2

A 9-month-old infant who failed to develop normally due to nutritional neglect developed secondary immunodeficiency characterized by marked thymic involution (atrophy or shriveling). The child died of systemic *P. aeruginosa* infection. Clinical manifestations included pneumonia, lung abscesses, and endocarditis. Multiple gangrenous ecthymas consisting of deep ulcers, inflammation, and induration were observed on the skin of the entire body. Autopsy revealed that the lungs were hemorrhagic and had multiple abscesses with necrotizing arteritis; the heart showed dark brown verrucae at the cusps of the mitral valve. Large numbers of *P. aeruginosa* were isolated from the lungs, heart, and skin lesions on bacteriologic examination. (Based on a case described by Ohshima et al., 1991.)

Questions:

1. How is the poor nutritional status of the infant related to development of secondary immunodeficiency and infection with *P. aeruginosa*? **A well-balanced diet is essential for optimal functioning of the immune system, which, in turn, is important in defense against infectious agents. *P. aeruginosa* infection in immunocompromised individuals can have devastating effects (as exemplified in this case history), whereas healthy individuals generally have no problem with these ubiquitous organisms. The fact that the malnourished infant had thymic atrophy is especially significant, since the thymus is the site of T lymphocyte maturation into immunocompetent cells.**

2. What is the cause of the widespread tissue destruction in the infant? ***P. aeruginosa* produces a large variety of extracellular enzymes and other factors that may contribute to tissue destruction and invasiveness. Exotoxin A, produced by approximately 90% of strains, is the most toxic substance that is synthesized by the organisms and is thought to play a major**

role in the disease process. The toxin inhibits protein synthesis by a mechanism that is identical to that of the fragment A portion of the toxin that is produced by *Corynebacterium diphtheriae*. It catalyzes the transfer of ADP-ribosyl of nicotinamide adenine dinucleotide (NAD) to a modified histidine residue on elongation factor 2 (EF-2) in eucaryotic cells. The ADP-ribosyl-EF-2 complex results in cessation of protein synthesis and cell death.**

3. Is the multisystem involvement unusual for *P. aeruginosa*? **Involvement of multiple organ systems is not unusual in immunocompromised individuals once *P. aeruginosa* infection has become established. The organisms can infect and proliferate in nearly all tissues and organs of the body. Organisms can become disseminated via the blood circulation and cause focal lesions distant from the original site of infection. They can also spread progressively to affect tissues surrounding a localized area of infection.**

Suggested Answers to

CASE STUDY 3

A 30-year-old man with quadriplegia due to spinal cord transection was transferred to a hospital from a chronic care facility because of fever (39.9°C temperature) and increased need for ventilatory support. The patient had ulcerative skin lesions ("bed sores") and had recently been given a 10-day course of intravenous oxacillin therapy. On presentation, his breath sounds in the left hemithorax were decreased. The white blood cell count was 12.0 × 10⁹/L; the differential showed increased percentages of segmented neutrophils and bands. Chest radiography revealed partial collapse of the left lung. Radiography after broncho-scopy indicated the presence of a persistent infiltrate in the left lower lobe. *B. catarrhalis* was cultured from the blood. Sputum cultures yielded *Acinetobacter anitratus, Klebsiella pneumoniae,* and *Haemophilus influenzae.* The patient improved during a 10-day course of ceftazidime therapy. (Based on a case described by Ioannis et al., 1995.)

Questions:

1. Is bacteremia due to *B. catarrhalis* unusual? **Bacteremia due to *B. catarrhalis* is relatively uncommon and has been documented mostly in individuals with significantly compromised host defenses. The organisms are usually associated with sinusitis, otitis media, and conjunctivitis, although bronchopulmonary infections are being reported with increasing frequency. *B. catarrhalis* is a member of the normal oropharyngeal flora.**

2. Which of the isolated organisms is most likely to be responsible for the pulmonary symptoms? **This is a question that cannot be answered without additional information, since all four of the organisms have been implicated in the etiology of pneumonia. Presence of an infiltrate in the left lower lobe of the lungs suggests that *B. catarrh-* *alis* may be involved, since these organisms are an important cause of lower respiratory tract infections. However, the other organisms cannot be excluded on this basis.**

3. What is the significance of the elevated white blood cell count and increased percentages of neutrophils? **Neutrophils are considered to be among the most important cells in host defense against bacterial infections. An increase in the number of these cells (and bands, which are immature neutrophils) can be detected in the peripheral blood circulation within one hour after infection with bacteria. They are the first cell type to be recruited to the site of infection within tissues. Neutrophils phagocytize, digest, and kill bacteria in a nonspecific manner.**

Answers to

Review Questions

1. A gram-negative rod is isolated from the sputum of a 20-year-old woman with cystic fibrosis. Laboratory tests reveal that the organism is an aerobic "nonfermenter" that produces a blue pigment and is highly resistant to numerous antibiotics. Given this description, the organism is MOST LIKELY to be:
   a. ***Pseudomonas aeruginosa***

2. Which of the following is an important factor in the virulence of *P. aeruginosa*?
   c. **Exotoxin A**

3. A factor produced by *P. aeruginosa* that can break down antibodies and complement is:
   d. **alkaline protease.**

4. Which of the following best describes the mechanism of action of exotoxin A?
   d. **It stops protein synthesis by ADP-ribosylation of elongation factor-2.**

5. *Pseudomonas* species are MOST LIKELY to cause serious infection in individuals who:
   d. **have a very low neutrophil count.**

6. Melioidosis is caused by which of the following organisms?
   b. ***Pseudomonas pseudomallei***

7. *P. aeruginosa* infection in patients with AIDS is MOST LIKELY to be manifested as:
   a. **pneumonia.**

8. Glanders is caused by which of the following organisms?
   d. ***Pseudomonas mallei***

CHAPTER 18

Vibrio and Other Curved Aerobic Gram-Negative Bacilli

Suggested Answers to

CASE STUDY 1: CHOLERA STRIKES DURING AIRPLANE FLIGHT

A businesswoman developed severe vomiting and diarrhea during a flight from Bangkok to Los Angeles. On landing she was examined at the airport clinic, but left against medical advice. Approximately 12 hours later she went into shock and was brought to an emergency room by concerned family members. The patient spent the next 4 days in the intensive care unit of the hospital. She had no recollection of dining in restaurants or eating seafood, except fried fish in Bangkok and sashimi on the airplane. Because of the short incubation period and lack of other in-flight cases, it seemed unlikely that the woman had become infected during the flight. Laboratory tests revealed that she had *V. cholerae*, serotype ogawa, biotype eltor in the stool. Outbreaks of cholera were reported in Bangkok and neighboring regions during the woman's visit. The patient was aware of possible dangers in drinking impure water, but not that this might give her cholera. (Based on a case reported in Los Angeles County Department of Health Services. [1994]. *Public Health Letter. 16(3), 1.*)

Questions:

1. Do most people become ill after consuming food or water that is contaminated with *V. cholerae*? **The majority (approximately 75%) of infections with *V. cholerae* are subclinical or relatively mild. There is a high incidence of individuals in endemic areas who have circulating antibodies and localized IgA specific for the cholera toxin and other antigens of the organisms, yet they have no history of having had cholera. Natural infection with *V. cholerae* induces a strong protective immune response against the organisms. In addition, it appears likely that some individuals may not get infected, since a large number of organisms must be consumed in order to overcome natural defense mechanisms in the upper gastrointestinal tract.**

2. Why did the woman go into shock? **Cholera is characterized by massive loss of fluid and electrolytes due to the action of the cholera toxin that is secreted by the organisms attached to the lumen of the small intestine.** As much as 20–30 liters of fluid can be lost within a 24-hour period, in striking contrast to the 250 ml that is normally passed in the stool. The effects of hypovolemic shock are seen in multiple organ systems, including the brain, heart, and kidneys.

3. What is the mechanism of action of the cholera toxin? **The cholera toxin consists of one A subunit and five B subunits. The B subunits bind to G_{M1} ganglioside on epithelial cells within the intestinal lumen. This allows passage of the A subunit into the cells and its cleavage into A1 and A2. The A1 subunit acts as an ADP-ribosyl transferase that moves ADP-ribose from NAD to Gs-alpha (a GTP-binding protein), resulting in permanent activation of adenylate cyclase and increased intracellular cAMP. The high level of cAMP, in turn, leads to open chloride channels in membranes and hypersecretion of isotonic fluid from the epithelial cells into the intestinal lumen.**

Suggested Answers to

CASE STUDY 2: WATERY STOOL IN COLLEGE STUDENT

A 20-year-old male college student arrived in an outpatient clinic complaining of severe abdominal pain and diarrhea. He stated that the episode began approximately 5 days previously as a mild stomachache. Two or three loose bowel movements per day began shortly thereafter. Forty-eight hours before his arrival in the clinic he began experiencing intermittent pain in the right lower quadrant of the abdomen that was increasing in severity. Physical examination revealed that he had a tender abdomen, normal vital signs, and no fever. The patient had not traveled out of the United States. In addition, he denied consuming raw seafood or drinking well water. His white blood cell count, platelet count, and hematocrit were within normal limits. Further laboratory evaluation revealed a watery stool that had a slightly greenish tinge and was negative for occult blood. However, numerous white blood cells were noted on microscopic examination of the fecal specimen. Cultures on SS agar and Hektoen agar were negative. A slender, curved gram-negative rod was eventually isolated on TCBS agar and Skirrow's medium incubated at 42°C under microaerophilic conditions. The typical darting motility of *Campylobacter* was observed with dark-field microscopy. Based on these findings a diagnosis of *Campylobacter jejuni* enteritis was made. Erythromycin was prescribed and the patient recovered promptly.

Questions:

1. What are the possible sources of infection with *C. jejuni*? **Animals (including chickens, turkeys, wild birds, swine, cattle, horses, dogs, and cats) are major reservoirs for human infection with *C. jejuni*. The organisms reside in the intestinal tract of healthy animals. In the United States, consuming and handling poultry products present the highest risk. Drinking contaminated water or raw milk can also lead to outbreaks. Human-to-human transmission can occur during oral-anal sexual activity.**

2. What are the characteristics of TCBS agar and Skirrow's medium that allowed the isolation of *C. jejuni*? **Skirrow's agar consists of a peptone and soy protein base supplemented with lysed horse blood. The medium also contains polymyxin B and trimethoprim, which inhibit the growth of many gram-negative enterics, and vancomycin, which prevents growth of gram-positive organisms. *C. jejuni*, however, is not inhibited by these antimicrobials. TCBS agar consists of a peptone base, yeast extract, sodium thiosul-**fate, citrate, bile salts, sucrose, and a bromthymol blue indicator. It is a commonly used selective and differential medium for vibrios and related organisms. Growth of *C. jejuni* was not obtained on SS and Hektoen agar because they contain combinations of chemicals (e.g., relatively high concentrations of bile salts, bromthymol blue, and acid fuchsin in the case of Hektoen agar) that are inhibitory. Furthermore, these two media are generally not incubated at 42°C under microaerophilic conditions, since they are used primarily for isolation of *Salmonella* and *Shigella*.**

3. Is enteritis due to *C. jejuni* common in the United States? ***C. jejuni* is thought to be the most common bacterial cause of enteritis in the United States and other developed countries. The highest incidence in the United States is seen in infants under the age of 1 year and in individuals between the ages of 15 and 29 years. Most cases are reported during the summer months.**

Suggested Answers to

CASE STUDY 3: PEPTIC ULCERS IN AN EXECUTIVE

A 50-year-old male executive of a large corporation repeatedly presented with epigastric discomfort, a burning sensation in the abdominal region, and indigestion with occasional bouts of nausea and vomiting. The symptoms were more pronounced after meals and consumption of alcohol, but were partially ameliorated by Pepto-Bismol. The patient experienced pain with gentle percussion over the midepigastric region. A gastric biopsy, obtained during endoscopy, was sent to the laboratory. A positive urease test was quickly obtained by using material from the biopsy specimen and a Warthin-Starry stain revealed the presence of spiral-shaped organisms. Small round colonies appeared within a week of incubation at 37°C in a microaerophilic environment on Skirrow's agar and Thayer-Martin agar. Oxidase and catalase reactions were positive, there was no growth at 25°C or 42°C, and nitrate reduction and hippurate hydrolysis tests were negative. A diagnosis of peptic ulcer disease due to *Helicobacter pylori* was made. A regimen of metronidazole, bismuth subsalycylate, and amoxicillin was prescribed. The patient's symptoms subsided and laboratory results from follow-up visits indicated that *H. pylori* had been eradicated.

Questions:

1. How is *H. pylori* able to survive the acidity of the stomach? **There are at least three mechanisms by which *H. pylori* is able to survive the acidity of the stomach: (a) it produces a powerful urease enzyme that breaks down urea, resulting in a protective "cloud" of ammonia that neutralizes the acidic environment; (b) it produces mucinase, which breaks down mucus, thus allowing the organisms to penetrate more easily to the epithelial side of the stomach, where there is much less acid; and (c) it produces a protease that alters the mucus layer so that it is less permeable to acids.**

2. Are there other bacteria that can survive in the stomach? **To date there is at least one other bacterium, *Gastrospirillum hominis* (also known as *H. heilmannii*), that is known to persist in the human stomach for extended periods of time. Recent genetic analyses indicate that the organism is similar to *Helicobacter felis*, which is found in the stomach of cats. *G. hominis* is a tightly spiraled, urease-producing organism that has up to 12 flagella at each pole. It is found in the parietal cell area of the stomach lining in approximately 1%–3% of humans. Its route of transmission is unknown. It is suspected that *G. hominis* will eventually be implicated in human disease, since it, like *H. pylori*, can induce inflammation.**

3. Is a combination of three drugs necessary to eradicate *H. pylori*? **Numerous trials have been conducted in the last few years to determine the optimal treatment for *H. pylori* infection. Many antimicrobial drugs with strong inhibitory action against the organisms in vitro have failed to be of clinical benefit, possibly because they are destroyed by gastric acidity or fail to penetrate into the mucous layer. Therapeutic regimens consisting of one or two drugs in various combinations have largely been unsuccessful. Recent studies indicate that triple therapy with a combination of metronidazole, a bismuth salt, and amoxicillin or tetracycline is effective in the great majority of cases.**

Answers to

Review Questions

1. Which of the following statements is correct for members of the *Vibrionaceae* family?
   a. **The majority of species cause severe diarrheal illness that requires prolonged treatment with combinations of antibiotics.**

2. A stool sample from a 46-year-old man with severe diarrhea is sent to the clinical laboratory for culture. The laboratory report indicates that the specimen contains oxidase-positive, gram-negative rods that form yellow colonies on TCBS agar and that they grow in medium containing 6% NaCl, but not in the presence of compound O/129. The organisms are MOST LIKELY to be:
   c. *Vibrio cholerae.*

3. Which of the following statements is correct regarding cholera toxin?
   b. **It is encoded by genes on plasmids.**

4. A potentially deadly organism that causes rapidly progressive and painful blister-like skin lesions is:
   d. *V. vulnificus.*

5. Skirrow's medium is used for:
   d. **selective isolation of *Campylobacter* and *Helicobacter*.**

6. The development of peptic ulcers is associated with which of the following organisms?
   a. *Helicobacter pylori*

7. Which of the following assays is useful is differentiating between *Campylobacter* and *Helicobacter*?
   c. **Urease test**

8. Disease produced by *Campylobacter jejuni* most closely resembles illness due to:
   b. *Salmonella* and *Shigella*.

CHAPTER 19
Gram-Negative Anaerobic Bacteria

Suggested Answers to

CASE STUDY 1: YOUNG WOMAN WITH ABDOMINAL PAIN

A 25-year-old woman complained of 3 days of diffuse abdominal pain. At first she thought the pain was cramps, but she was concerned because the pain persisted and she was losing her appetite. On physical examination she was febrile to 40°C, had an accelerated heart rate (155 beats/min), and a rapid respiratory rate. She had midgastric and right lower quadrant abdominal tenderness. Blood cultures obtained on admission were positive for anaerobic, gram-negative bacilli in 48 hours, at which time the patient was taken to surgery.

Questions:

1. What is the most likely group of anaerobes? **The most probable group is the *Bacteroides fragilis* group. The species most commonly associated with disease in humans is *Bacteroides fragilis*.**

2. The doctors decided to perform abdominal surgery. What types of diseases would you suspect could lead to anaerobic bacteremia? **Abdominal and pelvic abscesses, which in this case were secondary to appendicitis. Bowel perforation (cancer, trauma, etc.), obstruction, or improper blood flow can also** lead to anaerobic bacteremia with *B. fragilis* group organisms as well as other gastrointestinal tract flora.

3. What would tissue samples of the appendix probably grow on culture? **Most appendix abscesses are polymicrobial, involving anaerobic and aerobic bacteria representative of colonic contents. Therefore, one would expect multiple isolates, including *B. fragilis* group, *Clostridium* species, members of the *Enterobacteriaceae*, enterococci, etc.**

Suggested Answers to

CASE STUDY 2: ACUTE BACTERIAL CELLULITIS

A 58-year-old woman presented to the emergency department of a community hospital suffering from an acutely enlarged neck that was making it difficult for her to breathe. Onset was sudden, with no history of pharyngitis. Her condition worsened, and the doctors had to perform an emergency tracheotomy to keep her airway open. She was transported to the University Medical Center by air ambulance. On physical examination, she had massive swelling under her jaw and around her throat, most of which was bright red. There were no detectable fluid (pus) pockets to drain, so the physicians took some punch biopsies and started her on empiric antimicrobic therapy for acute cellulitis.

Questions:

1. What is your clinical diagnosis? Why is it important to establish that there was no previous history of sore throat? **Acute bacterial cellulitis. It is probably polymicrobial, involving anaerobes (*Fusobacterium* species, *Peptostreptococcus* species, and *Bacteroides* species), aerobes (*Viridans* group streptococci and group A streptococci), or both. Because the patient did not have a pharyngitis previously, Vincent's angina is less likely than Ludwig's angina.**

2. Aerobic cultures grew catalase-negative, gram-positive cocci exhibiting α-hemolysis. Anaerobic cultures grew indole-positive, gram-negative bacilli with rounded ends that were resistant to vancomycin and susceptible to kanamycin, colistin, and bile. Based on the clinical diagnosis and preliminary culture results, what are the most likely presumptive identifications? ***Viridans* group streptococci and *Fusobacterium* species, probably *F. necrophorum*.**

3. How does this patient's disease differ from Vincent's angina? Vincent's disease? **Vincent's angina usually begins with an anaerobic pharyngitis and/or peritonsillar abscess. This can progress to potentially fatal systemic disease (septic jugular vein thrombophlebitis, septicemia or Lemierre's syndrome, metastatic abscesses in the lungs). Vincent's disease, or trench mouth, is an acute (or chronic) ulcerative necrotizing gingivitis. This painful disease of the mouth and gums is also polymicrobial, involving *Fusobacterium* species and spirochetes.**

Answers to

Review Questions

1. Which genus consists of moderately saccharolytic, pigmented and nonpigmented, gram-negative organisms?
   a. *Prevotella*

2. Select the asaccharolytic, pigmented, nonspore-forming, gram-negative anaerobe(s) found in human infections due to animal bites.
   d. All of the above

3. Applying level II identification, which important test will help differentiate between *Porphyromonas* and *Prevotella?*
   b. Special potency disks, especially vancomycin

4. What wavelength is recommended when testing for fluorescence in anaerobic gram-negative pigmented organisms?
   c. Long

5. Which two enzymes are produced by strains of *B. fragilis,* and are easily detected in the laboratory?

   b.   Catalase, ß-lactamase

6. Which of the following media enhances the fluorescence test?

   d.   Lysed (laked) blood or rabbit blood agar

7. Why is it important to ensure special potency disks have warmed to room temperature before using them?

   d.   a and c are correct.

8. What obligate anaerobic gram-negative bacillus is described as long and thin with tapered ends, has no fluorescence, and is resistant only to vancomycin disks (susceptible to kanamycin, colistin, and 20% bile)?

   a.   *Fusobacterium nucleatum*

9. Which test differentiates the *B. ureolyticus* group from *Fusobacterium* species?

   b.   Nitrate

10. Special potency antimicrobial disks support level II identification of anaerobes by:

    a.   grouping organisms with similar characteristics (e.g., *B. fragilis* group).

CHAPTER 20

Gram-Positive Anaerobic Bacteria

Suggested Answers to

CASE STUDY 1: ALCOHOLIC WITH CHEST PAIN

A 63-year-old man presented to the emergency room with a chief complaint of localized right chest pain. Past medical history was unremarkable. Social history included homelessness, heavy smoker, and 2 to 3 glasses (pints) of wine daily. He denied intravenous drug abuse or sexually transmitted disease. He had received a tuberculosis skin test at the "shelter," and recalled it to be negative. Physical examination revealed poor dentition. His lungs were clear, but he winced in pain on deep inspiration. He had another tuberculin skin test, with an anergy panel, and was sent to x-ray. Chest radiographs indicated a mass in the right middle lobe near the rib cage. Closer inspection of his external chest revealed a 0.5-cm lesion that drained when pressure was applied.

Questions:

1. What organisms might cause this patient's symptoms? **Mycobacterium tuberculosis, Mycobacteria other than *Mycobacterium tuberculosis* (MOTT), *Nocardia* species, *Actinomyces* species, other oral aerobic and/or anaerobic flora (frequently polymicrobic), dimorphic fungi, *Cryptococcus neoformans*.**

2. What specimens would you send to the microbiology lab? What tests would you order? **Sputum smears for Gram stain and acid-fast stain. Sputum culture for aerobic (not anaerobic; see Chapter 24, Processing and Interpretation of Cultures from Clinical Specimens) bacteriology, mycobacteriology,** and mycology. Bronchoscopy specimens would be best (and you could add *Nocardia* and anaerobic studies if carefully collected and transported promptly). Additionally you would need a specimen from the draining sinus and an aspirate from the mass. Gram stain (look for sulfur granules), acid-fast stain, modified acid-fast stain, and calcofluor white stain for fungi. Culture for aerobic and anaerobic bacteria, mycobacteria, and fungi.

3. Gram-positive, delicately branching, club-end bacilli were seen in large clumps on drainage and aspirate specimens. Other stains were negative. What was the most likely organism? **Actinomyces species, often *A. israelii*.**

Suggested Answers to

CASE STUDY 2: SCHOOL TEACHER WITH FEVER

A 38-year-old female elementary school teacher went to her physician complaining of intermittent low-grade fever, weight loss over the last 6 months of 20 pounds, and abdominal discomfort. Initially she thought she had gotten the "bug that was going around," but her husband urged her to seek medical attention. A week prior to the current visit, she had a chest x-ray, purified protein derivative, urinalysis, and a stool specimen worked up for enteric or parasitic agents (including *C. difficile*), all of which were negative. Her fever was worse today, 39°C, and her doctor decided to admit her to the hospital. Admission labs were remarkable for a white cell count of 16,000 with 76% neutrophils. Blood cultures were drawn, and both anaerobic bottles were positive at 48 hours (aerobic bottles remained negative). Gram stain revealed gram-positive bacilli, and subculture produced a rapidly spreading anaerobic culture by the next day.

Questions:

1. What gram-positive anaerobes would one expect to see in blood cultures? **Most often they are contaminants (associated with venipuncture) belonging to the genera *Peptostreptococcus*, *Propionibacterium*, and even *Clostridium*. *Clostridium* species are involved in disease only about half the time they are isolated from blood.**

2. This spore-forming organism was saccharolytic (glucose, lactose, maltose, mannose) and proteolytic (hydrolyzes gelatin). Other than esculin hydrolysis, biochemical tests were negative. Using your tables, what identification do you propose? ***Clostridium septicum.***

3. What significance do you assign to this particular species? ***Clostridium septicum* bacteremia is closely associated with colorectal** carcinoma and sometimes is the primary presenting indicator of this malignancy. It is extremely important to convey the potential significance of these findings to the physician so that appropriate evaluation may proceed.

4. Under what circumstances would you expect *C. difficile* to cause abdominal discomfort and diarrhea? How is it diagnosed? **Following antimicrobial therapy, usually after 3 days of hospitalization (a 3-day incubation period exceeds expected onset of community-acquired infectious gastrointestinal disease). Disease can also present in an outpatient on oral antimicrobial therapy or home care. Diagnosis is usually by detection of toxin, either by cytotoxicity or antigen detection (EIA or latex agglutination).**

Answers to

Review Questions

1. Select the one best definition of an obligate anaerobe.
   b. **Fail to multiply in the presence of O_2 or in a CO_2 incubator**

2. The pathogenesis of gram-positive, nonspore-forming, anaerobic infections includes all of the following, EXCEPT:
   c. **always are toxin mediated.**

3. Characteristics of the *Peptostreptococcus* sp. include:
   d. **all of the above**

4. The most frequently isolated gram-positive, nonspore-forming bacilli is:
   d. ***Propionibacterium acnes.***

5. The most frequently isolated gram-positive spore-forming anaerobic pathogen is:
   b. ***Clostridium perfringens.***

6. Identify this isolate at level II: anaerobic gram-positive, nonspore-forming diphtheroid bacilli, nonmotile, and +/+/+ for catalase, indole, and nitrate, respectively.

    d. ***Propionibacterium acnes***

7. Identify this isolate at level II: gram-variable bacilli, Nagler positive, and –/+/–/+ for indole, nitrate, catalase, reverse CAMP, respectively.

    a. ***Clostridium perfringens***

8. Potential reactions on egg yolk agar include:

    d. **a and c only.**

9. The most potent biologic substance known is produced by which of the following bacteria?

    d. ***Clostridium botulinum***

10. *Clostridium difficile* toxins are often detected by which method?

    c. **Cytotoxicity assay**

CHAPTER 21

Mycobacteria

Suggested Answers to

CASE STUDY

A 32-year-old man presents with a low-grade fever, nonproductive cough, and a left upper lung lobe infiltrate 3 months after a diagnosis of AIDS. The patient's symptoms and radiograph improved, but 1 month later he was admitted with acute hepatitis. The usual antimycobacterial medications were administered but after the incident of hepatitis the medication was stopped. One year later, the same patient presented with fever, cough, and progression of his left upper lobe infiltrate. He improved after treatment for tuberculosis and 6 weeks later he was admitted with headache, fever, and a cough productive with purulent sputum.

Vital signs were: temperature, 40°C; pulse, 108 beats/min; respirations, 22/min; BP, 102/62. His general appearance was thin with minimal respiratory distress. Examination of his mouth revealed thrush and leukoplakia. A chest examination revealed bilateral inspiratory crackles over the upper lung fields.

Laboratory findings included white blood cell count, 4,800/μL; CD4 count, 5/μL. The findings in chemistry studies revealed aspartate transaminase, 50 U/L; alkaline phosphatase, 121 U/L. Bone marrow and sputum smears were positive for acid-fast bacilli. Lumbar puncture results were glucose, 43 mg/dL; protein, 50 mg/dL; white cell count, 10 cells/mm³ (all lymphocytes); India ink, negative; cryptococcal antigen titer, 1:32. A chest radiograph showed bilateral infiltrates.

Questions

1. What is the etiologic agent causing the recurrent respiratory symptoms? **Mycobacterium avium-intracellulare complex.**

2. What antimicrobial therapy would be appropriate? **This two-organism complex is resistant to most antituberculosis agents. Ansamycin and clofazimine are active against the complex and, if possible, should be used in combination with three other drugs (if three other drugs with activity can be found) to treat the infection.**

Answers to

Review Questions

1. A scotochromogen:
   b. **produces a yellow pigment only in the dark.**

2. Which of the following is not associated with *M. tuberculosis?*
   b. **DDS**

3. If more than 9 acid-fast bacilli are seen per microscopic field the report is:
   a. **greater than 9/field.**

4. The lepromatous form of leprosy is:
   d. **none of the above.**

5. A *Mycobacterium* is isolated and has the following characteristics: nonphotochromogen, produces a domed opaque yellow colony at 35°C and a transparent lobed buff colony at 25°C. The organism is most likely:

b.   *M. avium complex.*

6. An unknown *Mycobacterium* is positive for the nitrate test, both catalase tests, Tween 80 test, and may or may not be positive for the tellurite test; all other tests are negative including TCH. The organism is most likely:

d.   **none of these.**

CHAPTER 22
Spirochetes

Suggested Answers to

Eleven days after returning from a camping trip to the North Rim of the Grand Canyon (June 21, 1990), a 61-year-old man from California developed fever, chills, headache, myalgias, and drenching sweats. These symptoms lasted for 2 days. Over the next 2 weeks he experienced three febrile relapses and was finally hospitalized. A physical examination and a variety of laboratory tests were performed but were nondiagnostic. While in the hospital the patient experienced a fourth episode of fever during which time a peripheral blood sample was obtained and examined. Spirochetes were observed and relapsing fever was diagnosed. The patient was unable to recall a tick bite. He was treated with tetracycline and recovered.

After investigation of the cabin in which he stayed, and phone and mail surveys of over 10,000 other Grand Canyon visitors (from nine states, Canada, and Germany), 14 other cases (4 laboratory confirmed, 10 clinically defined) of relapsing fever were confirmed. The cabins were sprayed with an acaricide and structural changes were made to deter rodents from nesting in and around the buildings.

From: *Morbidity and Mortality Weekly Report.* (1991). *40* (18), 296–297.

Questions:

1. What is the most likely cause of this infection? *Borrelia recurrentis*

2. What three species cause endemic relapsing fever in the United States? *Borrelia parkeri, B. hermsii,* and *B. turicatate.*

3. What is the vector of epidemic relapsing fever? **The louse, *Pediculus humanus.***

Answers to

Review Questions

1. Which of the following techniques would be most appropriate for the diagnosis of Lyme disease?
   d. **There is no reliable test for Lyme disease at this time.**

2. A 9-year-old boy is admitted to the hospital after two bouts of fever (105°F), headache, myalgias, right upper quadrant pain, and chills. What is the most probable diagnosis and the likely drug of choice?
   c. **Relapsing fever, penicillin G**

3. Which of the following techniques is most appropriate for the identification of spirochetes in genital chancres?
   d. **Either b or c**

4. Infection of domestic animals with which of the following can result in significant economic losses?
   a. *Leptospira interrogans*

5. The successful treatment of syphilis is indicated by:
   b. **a reduction or elimination of the titer.**

6. *Treponema* species are transmitted to humans by which of the following?

   d. All of the above

7. The development of a maculopapular rash is characteristic of:

   c. secondary syphilis.

8. A pregnant woman is being treated with doxycycline for a spirochete infection. She is admitted to the hospital with headache and muscle pain and is going into labor in the first week of her seventh month of pregnancy. The above are characteristic of:

   a. the Yaws reaction.

9. Another name for the "bull's-eye" rash that is characteristic of Lyme disease is:

   d. erythema migrans.

10. Which of the following could result in a false-positive reaction for syphilis using a nontreponemal test?

   d. All of the above

CHAPTER 23

Chlamydia, *Mycoplasma*, and *Rickettsia*

Suggested Answers to

CASE STUDY: PRIMARY ATYPICAL PNEUMONIA IN A CHILD

A 12-year-old girl was admitted with fever, a persistent nonproductive cough, and night sweats; she appeared mildly dyspneic. Four weeks previously, the patient had been well. During the course of illness, she experienced episodic pain in the subscapular region and shoulder. On admission her vital signs were: temperature, 38.5°C; pulse 98/min; respirations, 29/min; and blood pressure, 125/65 mm Hg. Other laboratory tests indicated a leukocyte count of 6.3×10^9/L, white blood cell populations within normal limits, an increased blood sedimentation rate, and a high value for C-reactive protein. Chest radiographs showed bilateral lower lobe involvement. Blood cultures were negative and routine cultures of bronchial washings revealed no pathogens. An immunoblot for anti-I IgM was strongly positive and a complement fixation assay gave a serum antibody titer of >1:512 using *M. pneumoniae* antigen. Oral erythromycin and intravenous cefuroxime were administered. The patient turned afebrile within 2 days; improvement was slow, but uneventful. She was discharged from the hospital 5 days after admission.

Questions:

1. What does the strong positive for IgM antibodies suggest? **A possible parasite infection.**

2. Is a slow recovery typical for pneumonia due to *M. pneumoniae*? **No, usually the patient recovers rapidly.**

3. Is the patient immune to *M. pneumoniae* after this episode of illness? **No.**

Answers to

Review Questions

1. *Chlamydia trachomatis* is implicated in all of the following disease states, EXCEPT:
   d. **persistent unproductive cough.**

2. An adequate specimen for chlamydial isolation and identification should contain:
   d. **epithelial cells.**

3. Which of the following is NOT associated with *Chlamydia trachomatis*?
   b. **Iodine-negative intracytoplasmic inclusions**

4. Which of the following are the smallest microbes capable of cell-free reproduction?
   a. ***Mycoplasma* species**

5. Cold agglutinins that frequently appear following infection with *Mycoplasma pneumoniae* belong to which class of antibody?
   c. **IgM**

6. Which of the following organisms is MOST LIKELY to cause atypical pneumonia in a child?
   a. ***Mycoplasma pneumoniae***

7. Which of the following rickettsia can be cultivated on a cell-free medium?
   d. ***C. burnettii***

8. A patient presenting with a generalized papulovesicular rash, eschars, and a comment of association with wild rodents and *mite* bites is suspect of having:
   d. **Scrub typhus**

9. The organism *Coxiella burnetti* is the causative agent of:
   b. **Q fever.**

CHAPTER 24

Processing and Interpretation of Cultures from Clinical Specimens

Suggested Answers to

A 91-year-old male diabetic resident of a nursing home presented with a high fever, altered mental status, and severe soft tissue destruction at the site of what had been a minor skin lesion on his face. Two other patients in the nursing home had similar tissue destruction, one at the site of a surgical wound and one with no known prior wound or infection. During the same time period at the nursing home, three other patients had manifested various symptoms that could not be explained by their past medical histories, such as renal failure, hypotension, rash, and shock. One had died.

These patients suffered from invasive *Streptococcus pyogenes* disease (see Figure 24-9). Diabetes, old age, residence in nursing homes, and other underlying medical problems are all risk factors for this disease, which has an overall case fatality rate of 10% to 20%. It is possible to develop this disease without having a history of past streptococcal infection.

Invasive streptococcal disease is diagnosed by isolating *S. pyogenes* from a normally sterile site. Culture protocols must be designed such that this organism will be isolated, identified, and promptly reported.

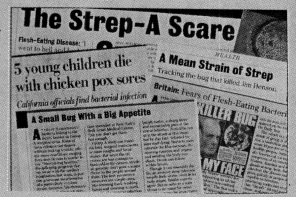

FIGURE 24-9 *Streptococcus pyogenes*, also known as group A *Streptococcus*, has received a lot of media attention in recent years.

Questions:

1. What is the most common infection caused by *S. pyogenes*? How is it diagnosed?
   S. pyogenes is most frequently associated with pharyngitis. Streptococcal pharyngitis can be diagnosed by isolating the organism in culture or by using rapid immunologic techniques to detect the presence of specific S. pyogenes antigens.

2. Describe some of the other severe diseases that can result following infection with this organism. **S. pyogenes can also cause scarlet fever (a severe form of pharyngitis that is caused by strains producing a potent toxin), rheumatic fever (a systemic disease that can result in permanent damage to the heart), glomerulonephritis (an inflammation of the** functional unit of the kidney, resulting in kidney dysfunction), and a form of toxic shock syndrome (a severe flu-like syndrome that can involve many organ systems, with up to 55% mortality).

3. Describe techniques that can be used to identify *S. pyogenes* in the laboratory. **S. pyogenes colonies are small, convex, and translucent, surrounded by a clear zone of ß-hemolysis. Gram stain of colonies would show gram-positive cocci or coccobacilli. To confirm the identification, catalase, PYR, and bacitracin susceptibility tests can be performed (catalase negative, PYR positive, bacitracin susceptible), and/or detection of the group A carbohydrate antigen can be performed.**

Answers to

Review Questions

1. Direct microscopic examination of clinical specimens offer the advantage of having results available much earlier than culture. What is one of the disadvantages of direct microscopic examination?

   c. **The results must be confirmed by culture.**

2. A gram-stained smear of an abscess specimen revealed numerous squamous epithelial cells, very few PMNs, numerous gram-negative rods, and numerous gram-positive and gram-negative cocci. Which is correct?

   a. **The specimen was probably not collected properly because there are so few PMNs.**

3. One suggested protocol for cerebrospinal fluid (CSF) culture includes blood agar, chocolate agar, and thioglycollate broth. Why does not this protocol include selective media such as MacConkey or Columbia colistin-nalidixic acid?

   c. **Because CSF does not ordinarily have normal flora, so there is no need to "select" for other types of organisms**

4. What type of information about the patient should the physician communicate to the laboratory when submitting specimens for culture?

   d. **All of the above**

5. Which of the following is NOT true about normal flora?

   b. **Normal flora usually causes a lot of trouble for the host, in the various sites in which they live.**

6. Which of the following is correct regarding presumptive and definitive identification?

   d. **Each laboratory needs to specify its own procedures defining when different types of isolates should be presumptively or definitively identified.**

7. Which of the following is NOT a means of detecting growth from any type of blood culture system?

   a. **Presence of PMNs in a Gram smear**

8. Which of the following is true of throat cultures?

   b. ***Neisseria gonorrhoeae,*** **which can cause pharyngitis, requires special selective media for isolation from throat specimens.**

9. Which of the following is NOT true of wound/abscess/soft tissue infections?

   a. **These infections are usually only caused by *Staphylococcus aureus.***

10. Which of the following is NOT true about reporting results?

    c. **Because most doctors have had training in infectious diseases, the laboratory can assume that all physicians fully understand all culture results and their significance.**

CHAPTER 25

Cerebrospinal Fluid and Other Body Fluids

Suggested Answers to

CASE STUDY

A 9-year-old girl was seen in the emergency room following the sudden onset of a seizure. Her temperature on admission was 107°F. Her CBC showed an increase in leukocytes and platelets. She was given Ativan for the seizures and Tylenol, cool mist, and ice packs for the fever. The patient had a ventriculoperitoneal (VP) shunt in place and a prior history of a brain tumor. Four days prior to admission, the patient experienced headaches associated with anorexia. The patient's condition worsened and she was given vecuronium, mannitol, and Decadron and was also treated with prophylactic antibiotic therapy. Blood and catheterized urine specimens were obtained prior to the administration of antibiotics. CSF obtained via her VP shunt showed a clear "ruddy-brown" colored fluid with a cell count of 88 leukocytes/µL and 4 red blood cells/µL, a glucose of < 20 mg/dL, and a total protein of > 300 mg/dL. Both blood and CSF cultures were positive for *Streptococcus pneumoniae*. Despite initiation of antibiotic therapy, the patient died 2 days later.

Questions:

1. What is the most probable diagnosis for this patient and why? **The most probable diagnosis is an acute meningitis, because of the sudden onset of symptoms (fever, seizures, headache), which rapidly progressed to death.**

2. What is the most probable cause of her condition? **A contaminated VP shunt is probably the most likely source of the CNS infection.**

3. Why was the patient given Decadron (dexamethasone) in addition to the antibiotic? **Antibiotics that destroy the bacterial cell wall cause the continued release of the organism's toxic components, continuing the effects of the body's immune response to infection. Use of adjunctive therapy with dexamethasone and other corticosteroids with antibiotics helps to reduce the intensity of the immune response.**

Answers to

Review Questions

1. What are the three most common pathogens of acute meningitis?
    c. ***S. pneumoniae, H. influenzae, N. meningitidis***

2. CSF taken from a febrile 1-day-old infant showed gram-positive cocci in singles, pairs, and chains. The most likely organism would be:
    a. ***S. agalactiae.***

3. CSF taken from an elderly diabetic woman had an increased protein level, a low glucose level, 1,000 PMNs/µL, and no organisms seen on the Gram stain. The most likely organism would be:
    d. ***S. pneumoniae.***

4. Complications of pneumonia include:
    d. **both a and c.**

5. Body fluid infections arise from:
    d. **all of the above.**

6. Which statement below is FALSE concerning the collection of sterile body fluid samples?

   d. **Avoid anticoagulant due to its inhibiting properties to some organisms. If an anticoagulant must be used, use EDTA.**

7. An elderly man with fever, cough, and dyspnea was seen in the emergency room. The patient was diagnosed with pneumonia. Purulent pleural fluid was collected and sent to the laboratory. The Gram stain showed gram-negative pleomorphic rods. What is the most likely organism?

   a. *Bacteroides*

8. Which of the following statements is FALSE concerning clinical symptoms of CNS infections?

   b. **Symmetrical petechial rash is seen in *Haemophilus* infections.**

9. A 65-year-old man visited his physician complaining of a headache increasing in severity, nausea, vomiting, and changes in mood for the past month. What course of action should be taken?

   b. **Perform a computed tomography scan immediately to rule out a CNS abscess.**

10. Which statement is FALSE concerning the pathogenesis of meningitis?

    c. **Once inside the CNS, the organisms must overcome the abundant white blood cells, complement, and antibodies in the CSF.**

CHAPTER 26
Blood Cultures

Suggested Answers to

Mr. Smith, a 42-year-old construction worker, cut his thumb while demolishing part of a building. By the next day the area around the cut was red and the thumb was sore, but he endured the pain as he worked all day. By evening, the thumb was swollen and throbbing, with some yellowish white material oozing out, and he noticed red streaks going up the inside of his forearm. He suddenly began to have a shaking chill and felt queasy, so his wife drove him to the hospital emergency room. On arrival at the emergency room his temperature had reached 39.7°C. He was flushed and appeared ill, with a pulse of 125 and a blood pressure of 100/60, compared to his usual of 145/85.

Blood cultures were drawn, and Mr. Smith was started on intravenous fluids and antibiotics. After about 8 hours of incubation, there was a positive blood culture signal on the instrument, and medium-large cocci in small groups and single were seen on the Gram stain. By morning he was not improved. Methicillin resistance was determined and the antibiotic was changed in the evening. By the next morning he was somewhat better, and his subsequent recovery over the next few days was uneventful.

Questions:

1. What were the most likely causes of the symptoms presented at the emergency room? **From the signs and symptoms, such as swelling, redness, pus production, and red streaks on the arm, it appeared that he had a bacterial infection. The most likely etiologic agents were *Streptococcus pyogenes*, *Staphylococcus aureus*, or possibly an enteric gram-negative bacillus or common environmental contaminant.**

2. Describe how the blood culture specimens should have been collected (when to collect, how much blood, etc.). **Two blood culture sets should be collected immediately following the physician's decision to perform a blood culture. Prepare the venipuncture site on one arm by using the typical alcohol and iodine disinfection procedure. Collect 20 to 30 mL of blood and divide the blood equally between two culture bottles, thus providing about a 1:10 ratio of blood to broth. Repeat the same disinfection and collection procedure for the other arm.**

3. What is the most likely presumptive identification of the pathogen, and what rapid tests could have been used to identify this organism? **Based on the percentage likelihood and cell morphology seen on the Gram stain, it is more likely that the organism is *Staphylococcus* than *Streptococcus*. Rapid tests such as catalase, coagulase, or PYR, which could be performed after centrifugation of about 10 mL of culture broth, would be useful in determining a presumptive identification. Definitive identification should come from complete testing of colonies that grow on the agar media.**

Suggested Answers to

CASE STUDY 2: ENDOCARDITIS CHALLENGE

A 35-year-old woman with a history of childhood rheumatic fever underwent excessive dental work without antimicrobial prophylaxis. About 2 weeks later she was examined in a neighborhood clinic because of fatigue, various muscle and joint aches, nonproductive cough, and low-grade fever. A radiograph of her chest did not reveal the etiology of these signs and symptoms, and tests for rheumatoid arthritis and tuberculosis were negative. About 10 mL of blood drawn from her right arm and inoculated into an aerobic blood culture bottle resulted in the recovery of a few colonies of what appeared to be a staphylococcus skin contaminant.

About 3 weeks after the original examination, she returned with the same signs and symptoms as previously. Repeat examination demonstrated the original findings plus an enlarged heart, bilateral pleural effusions, and weight loss. At this time the patient was admitted to the hospital having a temperature of 38.1°C and small "splinter hemorrhage" on one finger. A cardiac examination showed rapid heart rate and heart murmur. An echocardiogram demonstrated mitral valve regurgitation. Each of five sets of blood cultures taken over 24 hours from each arm was positive with α-hemolytic, gram-positive cocci.

Questions:

1. Why was there clinical evidence of endocarditis in the original episode, but not "positive" blood cultures? (What should have been done differently during the original examination to recover and identify the agent of possible endocarditis?) **The volume of blood collected was too small to ensure recovery of sparse numbers of bacteria in the blood stream. Since blood was collected from only one arm, it would be difficult to determine whether this was a contaminant or a pathogen. Collection of two or three blood culture sets of 20 to 30 mL each from at least two different body sites would have greatly improved the likelihood of recovering a pathogen, as well as assisting in differentiating between an infection and contamination.**

2. What role did the dental work play in causing the endocarditis. **Because rheumatic fever creates a preexisting risk of endocarditis, resulting from bacteria colonizing on damaged heart tissue, an antimicrobic is often administered before dental surgery. During dental work, bacteria can enter the blood stream via the capillaries around the teeth and gums and colonize on the damaged heart tissue and further damage the heart valves.**

3. What is the most likely microbial pathogen causing this problem? **Based on the percentage likelihood of causes of endocarditis under these circumstances, the observation of gram-positive cocci, and the growth of α-hemolytic colonies, the infection is most likely caused by alpha streptococci (viridans streptococci).**

Answers to

Review Questions

1. The presence of viable bacteria in the bloodstream is referred to as:
   b. **bacteremia.**

2. The type of bacteremia that occurs when bacteria periodically enter the bloodstream from an established abscess is:
   c. **intermittent.**

3. A blood culture medium that would NOT be appropriate for the recovery of aerobic bacteria would be:
   d. **thioglycollate broth with 5% carbon dioxide.**

4. Which of the following is most significant in recovering clinically significant isolates from blood cultures?
   a. **Scrub the venipuncture site with alcohol and iodine compounds.**

5. The BACTEC fluorescent system and the BacT/Alert blood culture system detect bacterial growth in the bottle by:

   c. **carbon dioxide production detected by a photodetector.**

6. A conventional broth blood culture system has incubated for 12 hours since it was collected. Which of the following procedures should be performed at this time (nothing except incubation has been performed up to this time)?

   b. **Gram stain and blind subculture**

7. Which of the following are two of the most predominant etiologic agents of bacteremia?

   d. ***Staphylococcus aureus* and *Escherichia coli***

8. One blood culture set was collected from each of the patient's arms. At 24 hours, one bottle of each set produced growth of a gram-positive coccus in clusters. Which of the following is the best interpretation?

   a. **This bacterium is probably a clinically significant isolate.**

9. For optimal recovery of bacteria from blood cultures from an adult, collect _____.

   c. **20 to 30 mL of blood and divide it between two culture bottles**

10. One of the reasons most blood culture media contain sodium polyanetholsulfonate (SPS) is because that chemical:

    d. **inactivates certain antimicrobics.**

CHAPTER 27
The Respiratory Tract

Answers to

Review Questions

1. One of the most common problems associated with the collection of samples for the diagnosis of upper respiratory tract infections is that:
   b. **a wide variety of normal flora accompanies the sample.**

2. Which of the following would be reason to reject a sample collected for diagnosis of streptococcal pharyngitis?
   e. **All of the above.**

3. Cystine-tellurite blood agar is especially useful in the diagnosis of infection with *Corynebacterium diphtheriae* because:
   d. **colony morphology of the organism is more diagnostic on this media.**

4. The specimen of choice for the diagnosis of whooping cough is a:
   a. **nasal pharyngeal wash or swab.**

5. Colonies of *Staphylococcus* can easily be differentiated from colonies of *Streptococcus* by a(n):
   b. **catalase test.**

6. Respiratory tract samples that are suspected to contain *Neisseria gonorrhoeae* should only be transported in a standard Ames system if:
   c. **activated charcoal is added.**

7. *Neisseria gonorrhoeae* should always be tested for sensitivity to:
   c. **penicillin.**

8. Methicillin-resistant *Staphylococcus aureus* is not sensitive to:
   d. **All of the above**

9. When grown on chocolate agar incubated in carbon dioxide *Moraxella catarrhalis* may sometimes be confused with:
   a. *Haemophilus influenzae.*

10. Which of the following specimen collection techniques should be reserved for very few situations . . . and why?
    e. **Both a and b**

CHAPTER 28
Ear, Eye, and Sinus Tracts

Suggested Answers to

A 24-year-old man was found by his ophthalmologist to have keratitis. He wore soft contact lenses. The doctor obtained specimens by corneal scrapings, biopsy, and keraplasty. All specimens were sent to the laboratory and distributed to the microbiology and histopathology areas for testing. The man's contact lenses, lens storage case, and home water supply were all examined for microorganisms. From the corneal tissue samples, no pathogenic bacteria, fungi, or viruses were recovered. Organisms were observed using light and electron microscopy, but immunochemical staining was not helpful. Viable organisms were recovered from the corneal biopsy specimen. A wide range of organisms was found in the lens storage case. One of these organisms was associated with the contact lens. After prolonged culture the organism was recovered.

Questions:

1. What causative organism most likely caused the patient's keratitis? **The amoeba and acanthamoeba.**

2. Which stains would you suggest for the corneal scrapings? **Giemsa stain, the corneal scraping.**

3. This organism can cause keratitis and blindness. What steps would you suggest to contact lens wearers to avoid such serious problems? **Follow the contact lens manufacturer's directions for disinfection of contact lenses, use heat disinfection to kill cysts reliably, do not wear contact lenses overnight or while swimming.**

Answers to

Review Questions

1. The majority of the sinuses around the nose naturally drain by means of:
   b. **gravity.**

2. Organisms routinely found in the eye include:
   a. **coagulase-negative staphylococci and diphtheroids.**

3. When culturing ear infections, the pathogen most likely to be isolated is:
   c. *Pseudomonas aeruginosa.*

4. Acute otitis media (AOM) is most likely found in which age group?
   a. **Toddlers**

5. A complication of sinus infections can be:
   d. **brain abscesses.**

6. Inflammation of the cornea can be caused by bacteria, mycobacteria, fungi, parasites, or viruses. When a yeast causes keratitis it is most likely:
   b. *Candida albicans.*

7. The most serious ocular infection is _____. The reason for medical concern is the risk of blindness without a quick identification of the organisms and treatment.

   c. endophthalmitis

8. The doctor would make the diagnosis of AOM by examining the:

   c. condition of the tympanic membrane.

9. There are noncultural detection methods for organisms from the eyes, ears, and sinus tracts. These methods can be helpful in confirming the identification when antimicrobial treatment may have started before the specimens for culture were obtained. An example of a nonculture method is:

   b. enzyme-linked immunosorbent assay.

10. With the changes in recreation and in advances in eye care, new diseases of the ear and eye are being seen. These conditions of the 1990s include all, EXCEPT:

    c. coagulase-negative staphylococci on the eye.

CHAPTER 29

The Urinary Tract

Suggested Answers to

CASE STUDY

A 30-year-old woman came to the emergency room complaining of a 2-day history of fever, chills, dysuria, and back pain. Her history indicated several similar episodes within the past 15 years. STAT urinalysis indicated increased protein, blood, and WBCs in the urine. The patient, who was also 37 weeks' pregnant, was admitted into the hospital. The patient was started on a 72-hour course of IV cefazolin.

The laboratory reported that the patient's urine had more than 100,000 cfu/mL of *E. coli*. The symptoms of her UTI resolved with treatment. She was discharged with a 10-day course of cephalexin, followed by a 30-day course of nitrofurantoin.

Questions:

1. Based on the symptoms of the patient, what type of UTI did she have? **The patient had the classic symptoms of pyelonephritis.**

2. The physician put the patient on prolonged antimicrobial treatment after her symptoms resolved. Discuss why this might have been done. **The patient had a history of recurrent UTI. This may indicate a complicated UTI, in which pathogens adhere to an internal sur-** **face or structure of the patient's urinary tract. This promotes recurrence. Very often, these bacteria have developed antimicrobial resistance. Prolonged treatment is used to clear these bacteria from protected niches.**

3. What are the most common uropathogens associated with this type of UTI? **Pyelonephritis is usually caused by a member of the Enterobacteriaceae or *S. aureus*.**

Answers to

Review Questions

1. Which of these cannot be submitted for culture to diagnose UTI?
   b. Foley catheter tips

2. Which of the following are accepted methods for preserving bacterial counts in urine before laboratory processing?
   d. All are acceptable.

3. Which of the following best describes pyelonephritis?
   c. Fever, flank pain, combined with lower urinary tract symptoms.

4. Each of the following describes complicated urinary tract infections EXCEPT:
   b. primarily associated with young, sexually active females.

5. Urinary tract infections are more common in women than in men because:

   d.   **a and c are true.**

6. Which of the following collection methods will likely result in the best specimen from a 6-month-old child?

   a.   **Suprapubic aspirate**

7. Acute urethral syndrome:

   c.   **may cause symptoms consistent with urethritis or cystitis.**

8. Many laboratories use >100,000 cfu/mL to define significant bacteriuria in:

   a.   **clean-catch midstream urine from asymptomatic patients.**

9. Asymptomatic bacteriuria:

   b.   **is a risk to pregnant women.**

10. Which is NOT a virulence factor for uropathogenic *E. coli*?

    b.   **Flagellum**

CHAPTER 30
The Genital Tract

Suggested Answers to

CASE STUDY

A 26-year-old woman was seen in the emergency department with complaints of a painful left shoulder and left knee. She was nauseous and had vomited several times in the past 48 hours. On physical examination she had restricted motion in her shoulder and her left knee was hot and swollen. She was also noted to have a thick vaginal discharge. Her temperature was 39°C; her white blood cell count was elevated at 16,000/mm^3. She had a history of having several sexual partners. Cultures and Gram stains were ordered on vaginal secretions and joint fluid. Gram stains showed numerous polymorphonuclear leukocytes. Although no bacteria were seen on smear, both the vaginal and joint fluid cultures grew the causative agent. After the diagnosis was made, tests for HIV were ordered.

Questions:

1. What is your diagnosis of this patient's infection? What is the association between the vaginal discharge and painful shoulder and knee? **The patient likely has a sexually transmitted disease. The sexually transmitted pathogen most likely to cause joint inflammation is *Neisseria gonorrhoeae*. This patient has septic arthritis, a complication of gonorrhea.**

2. Why was HIV testing ordered? **The patient's history of having several sexual partners** makes her a potential risk for HIV infection. Simultaneous infection with HIV frequently occurs with other sexually transmitted pathogens.

3. Why would there be added concern if this patient were pregnant? **Neonatal conjunctivitis (ophthalmia neonatorum) due to infection with *N. gonorrhoeae* may be acquired during birth. The use of silver nitrate or antibiotics placed in infants' eyes at birth has resulted in a considerable decline in incidence of this infection.**

Answers to

Review Questions

1. A potential source of infection in the female peritoneal cavity is:
   b. bacteria entering the body through the vagina.

2. The vulva refers to:
   b. the female external genitalia.

3. The resident flora of the female genital tract varies with:
   d. two of the above (a and b)

4. The predominant microorganisms found in the healthy vagina of adult women are:
   c. lactobacilli.

5. The most common female gynecologic complaint is:
   c.   **vaginal discharge.**

6. The following microorganism may be associated with neonatal sepsis and meningitis:
   d.   *Streptococcus agalactiae.*

7. The microorganism most closely associated with bacterial vaginosis is:
   c.   *Gardnerella vaginalis.*

8. The microorganism that may cause neonatal conjunctivitis is:
   a.   *Neisseria gonorrhoeae.*

9. The encapsulated, gram-negative bacterium that causes donovanosis is:
   d.   *Calymmatobacterium granulomatis.*

10. An example of a serologic assay to detect "treponemal" antibodies is the:
    b.   **FTA-ABS test.**

11. Microorganisms most often associated with pelvic inflammatory disease include:
    d.   **two of the above (a and c)**

12. A disease characterized by painful, necrotizing, ulcerative lesions (often called "kissing" lesions) at the site of inoculation is:
    b.   **chancroid.**

13. A cytobrush is often used to obtain cells for culture in the diagnosis of infection with:
    a.   *Chlamydia trachomatis.*

14. Which organism has been associated with PID, but which also may cause infertility, premature labor, and spontaneous abortion?
    d.   *Mycoplasma hominis*

15. Certain toxigenic strains of which organism, initially linked to tampon use, may cause toxic shock syndrome?
    b.   *Staphylococcus aureus*

CHAPTER 31
The Gastrointestinal Tract

Suggested Answers to

CASE STUDY

A blood culture, wound culture, and fecal culture are requested on a 56-year-old man in the emergency department (ED). On checking his order in the computer, you notice that his liver function tests are all abnormal. The ED nurse calls the microbiology laboratory and says the man had been fishing yesterday in a salt-water estuary and was hooked in the arm by the fishhook. He came to the ED after complaining of nausea and vomiting and fever.

Questions:

1. What organism do you suspect? ***Vibrio vulnificus.***

2. What culture protocol should be initiated to ensure recovery of this organism? **In addition to the usual fecal isolation media, inoculate a TCBS plate and an alkaline peptone broth. The wound protocol should also include TCBS in addition to the usual media.**

3. In addition to salt-water estuaries, what are other sources of infection with this organism?

***Vibrio vulnificus* is found in salt water, brackish water, and shellfish (especially oysters). Drinking contaminated water or eating contaminated oysters is another source of infection.**

4. Why did this patient have the complication of septicemia? **The patient has underlying liver disease, which predisposes to more severe infections with *Vibrio vulnificus*.**

Answers to

Review Questions

1. Which of the following is an appropriate isolation media for the organism listed?
   d. Enteropathogenic *Escherichia coli*— Sorbitol-MAC

2. What medium is appropriate for isolation of *Campylobacter* species?
   a. Skirrow's medium

3. Of the following which would require rejection of a fecal specimen?
   c. Feces mixed with urine

4. What organism causes GI infections due to overgrowth in diabetic or immunocompromised patients?
   b. *Candida albicans*

5. *Shigella* infections, common in day-care centers, are transmitted from person to person most often because of:

   d.   none of the above

6. What part of the GI flora has the largest amount of normally occurring flora?

   c.   Lower

7. What enrichment broth is recommended for isolation of *Vibrio* species?

   a.   Alkaline peptone broth

8. Gram stain of a fecal sample is useful for:

   b.   enumeration of WBCs.

9. Which of the following is considered highly selective media in the isolation of *Salmonella* and *Shigella*?

   c.   Brilliant green agar

10. Which of the following organisms must be incubated at 25°C to ensure recovery from fecal specimens?

    a.   *Yersinia*

CHAPTER 32
Skin Infections

Suggested Answers to

A 40-year-old Hispanic woman was seen for a chronic draining wound and an abnormal chest film. The patient was in excellent health until 4 to 5 months previous to being seen, when she was struck by her right scapula by a refrigerator door. One to 2 months later she noted a raised pustule over the area in question. The patient was seen by her primary care physician who opened the lesion and prescribed ciprofloxacin. Over the next month she noticed what she felt were some bone fragments coming from this site as well as clear fluid. An x-ray done of the chest and scapula revealed possible osteomyelitis of the right scapula and an abnormal left chest. The patient was referred to both an orthopedic surgeon and a pulmonologist.

The orthopedic surgeon did initial debridement and culture. *P. acnes* was initially grown and the patient was placed on high-dose penicillin. The wound did not heal and presented to the infectious disease specialist as a fistula with surrounding discoloration. Specimens were obtained for culture.

Questions:

1. Imagine you are the microbiologist tasked with the responsibility of culturing these specimens. What organisms would you suspect might be responsible for this infection? **Since an anaerobic organism (*Propionibacterium acnes*) had previously been isolated from this patient, it is important to do appropriate cultures to see if this organism is still present. The presence of a fistula means that a focus of infection in deeper tissues is present, and anaerobic bacteria are often present in these types of infections. Also, cultures should be adequate to isolate common aerobic agents of wound infections such as staphylococci, streptococci, and gram-negative bacilli. A key with this patient is that she had an abnormal chest film, which would lead one to suspect that the fistula was draining a lung infection. Therefore, it is important to culture for *Mycobacteria*, systemic fungi, and *Nocardia*. *Mycobacterium tuberculosis* was isolated from this patient.**

2. What is the significance of *P. acnes* in this case? ***Propionibacterium acnes* is a part of the normal flora of the skin. Although it can cause infection, particularly in immunocompromised patients, it is likely in this case that it was a skin contaminant. It is much faster growing than *M. tuberculosis*, which caused it to appear as the only isolate on initial culture.**

Answers to

Review Questions

1. Which of the following are part of the normal flora of the skin?
   b.   Corynebacteria and *Staphylococcus epidermidis*

2. What are the best specimens to obtain for culture of skin lesions?
   d.   Aspirate from a closed abscess or tissue

3. Opportunists generally invade the skin through:
   b.   breaks in the skin.

4. What are the most common bacterial agents of skin and wound infections?
   c.   *Staphylococcus aureus, Streptococcus pyogenes,* and anaerobic bacteria

5. Which bacteria commonly cause impetigo?
   a.   *Streptococcus pyogenes* and *Staphylococcus aureus*

6. What is the skin infection caused by *Erysipelothrix rhusiopathiae* called?
   d.   Erysipeloid

7. Which description fits *Bacillus anthracis?*
   b.   Gram-positive, spore-forming bacillus

8. What is the most common cause of actinomycosis in humans?
   b.   *Actinomyces israelii*

9. Skin infections with severe systemic manifestations that include desquamation (peeling) of the skin include which of the following?
   a.   Toxic shock syndrome and scalded skin syndrome

10. Material from an infected dog bite wound was Gram stained. Microscopic examination of the stained smear showed gram-negative coccobacilli. What is the most likely organism that will be isolated?
   b.   *Pasteurella multocida*

CHAPTER 33
Deep Tissues and Internal Organ Sites

Suggested Answers to

A 53-year-old man with leukemia who has recently undergone bone marrow transplantation (BMT) presents with abdominal pain and fevers. His post-BMT course had been complicated by fevers, neutropenia, an upper gastrointestinal bleed, and a central venous catheter infection. He had received antibiotics, and with a return of his leukocytes, improved. It is now 1 month later. He has noticed fevers to 101°F and vague abdominal discomfort. A liver ultrasound shows a collection of fluid in the left lobe of the liver.

Questions:

1. What is the diagnosis? **Liver abscess.**

2. List the possible pathogenic organisms that might be involved. **The list is almost endless. It includes any of the normal gastrointestinal flora, including anaerobes (*Bacteroides, Peptostreptococcus, Fusobacterium*, etc.); facultative aerobes, most commonly *Staphylococcus aureus* and the coagulase-negative staphylococci; *Enterococcus* species; the Enterobacteriaciae, with *Escherichia coli* being the most common gram-negative bacillus isolated; and numerous other gram-positive and gram-negative bacteria. Because of this patient's immunocompromised state, yeasts (especially *Candida* species) must also be considered. The molds would be unlikely, and the mycobacteria, amoebae, parasites, and other unusual organisms would be extremely rare causes of a liver abscess.**

3. What recommendations will you give the clinicians when they ask you how to submit the aspirated material? **You should recommend that a large amount of pus in a sterile syringe (with needle removed!) or other closed container be submitted to your laboratory immediately after obtaining the specimen from the patient. Special anaerobic transport media can be utilized if desired, but if the amount of pus is large, and the syringe has no extra air in it or the sterile container is brought immediately to your laboratory, then anaerobic swabs and transport media are not mandatory. Swabs alone may be adequate for submission if several are submitted and only bacteria are suspected, but swabs should not be used when submitting requests for fungal, mycobacterial, or other special handling. The clinician should request bacterial stains (Gram stain), along with aerobic and anaerobic bacterial cultures. If the patient had any previous or current evidence of fungal or mycobacterial infection, then fungal stain and culture, as well as mycobacterial stains and cultures, should also be requested.**

Answers to

Review Questions

1. What would be the most likely Gram stain finding in a specimen obtained from a patient with a pancreatic abscess following cholecystitis (infection in the bile ducts)?
   c. **Many white blood cells, moderate gram-negative bacilli, moderate gram-positive cocci**

2. The most common cause of osteomyelitis is:
   b. *Staphylococcus aureus.*

3. You receive a specimen from the neurosurgical operating room labeled "brain abscess." No other clinical information is given. What is the minimum processing that this specimen requires?
   b. **Gram stain, fungal stain, culture for aerobic and anaerobic bacteria, and fungi**

4. The medical student from the HIV ward brings a specimen labeled "lymph node aspirate" to your lab for processing. The patient has fevers, weight loss, a cough with bloody sputum, and two other enlarged cervical lymph nodes. What is the minimum processing that this specimen requires?
   c. **Gram stain, fungal stain, mycobacterial stain, culture for aerobic and anaerobic bacteria, fungi and mycobacteria**

5. When a deep tissue infection in the abdomen is cultured, what group of organisms is most commonly found in polymicrobic infections?
   d. **Anaerobes**

6. The single most common organism isolated from deep tissue infections is:
   a. *S. aureus.*

7. Which tissue is *M. tuberculosis* least likely to infect?
   d. **Brain**

8. Which of the following is considered to be a common pathogenic (not opportunistic) cause of human deep tissue infections?
   d. *Clostridium perfringens*

9. Which of the following is considered to be an opportunistic cause of human deep tissue infections?
   b. *E. coli*

10. You perform a Gram stain on a tissue sample submitted for routine bacterial studies and labeled "peritoneum." You document many white blood cells and no bacteria, but see many budding yeastlike cells. What is your next course of action?
    a. **In addition to inoculating standard aerobic and anaerobic media, inform the clinician of your findings and bring any remaining specimen to the fungal lab for special stains and plating.**

CHAPTER 34

Basic Concepts and Techniques in Mycology

Answers to

Review Questions

1. The drug amphotericin B interferes with permeability of the fungus cell wall because of its affinity for which substance in the cell wall?
   c. **Ergosterol**

2. All except which of the following are characteristic of fungi?
   b. **Chlorophyll**

3. Which of the following criteria are used to classify fungi into phyla?
   c. **Sexual spore type**

4. Which of the following is a sexual spore?
   d. **Zygospore**

5. Which of the following best stains fungal elements in smears for detail?
   d. **Periodic acid-Schiff**

6. The hypha pictured in Figure 34-6 is:
   a. **septate.**

7. Sporangiospores are typical of which group of fungi?
   a. **Zygomycetes**

8. No sexual spores have been identified for members of the class:
   d. ***Deuteromycota.***

9. Which of the following is associated with conidia production?
   c. **Phialide**

10. A bud coming off a parent cell is called a:
    b. **blastoconidium.**

CHAPTER 35

Collection and Processing of Fungal Specimens

Suggested Answers to

A 15-year-old boy injured his eye when a friend struck him in the face with a twig. Over the next few days he developed an ulcer and cloudiness in his cornea associated with some decrease in vision. His ophthalmologist suspected a fungal infection, and submitted corneal scrapings to the laboratory.

Questions:

1. What is the first thing you should do with the specimen after receiving it in the mycology laboratory? **The specimen should be divided into one portion for KOH prep and one portion for culture on fungal media if sufficient specimen is received. If there is insufficient specimen, direct exam in** *sterile* **saline on a** *sterile* **slide can be performed first; then the specimen can be transferred to culture media.**

2. What media should be planted? **Under most circumstances, one would expect saprophytic molds to cause corneal infections following injury to the eye. Therefore, a good general fungal medium such as Sabouraud's agar should be inoculated. If sufficient specimen is available, inhibitory agars should be inoculated to reduce bacterial contamination.**

3. Under what conditions should it be incubated? **In general, the cultures should be incubated at ambient room air conditions.**

4. What would you expect to see on the direct examination with KOH? **If the infection is a mycotic keratitis (corneal fungal infection), one would expect to see fungal hyphae in direct KOH preparations.**

Answers to

Review Questions

1. The function of 15% KOH in the direct examination of skin, hair, and nail scrapings is to:
   c. **clear and dissolve debris.**

2. All of the following are commonly used methods for the microscopic examination of filamentous molds, EXCEPT:
   b. **Gram stain.**

3. A medium appropriate for use in making a slide culture preparation is:
   b. **potato dextrose agar**.

4. India ink is useful for the microscopic demonstration of:
   c. **capsules.**

5. One of the better media for routine isolation of fungi is:
   a. **Sabouraud's dextrose agar**.

6. Which of the following is most often used to prepare a slide from a tease prep of a plate culture for microscopic observation of a dermatophyte?
   a. **Lactophenol cotton blue**

7. In which of the following specimens is it important to perform a direct examination for fungi in addition to setting up a fungal culture?
   d. **All of the above**

8. Which of the following would be expected to have moist, creamy or glabrous colonies?
   d. **Yeasts**

9. A slide culture is useful to demonstrate which of the following?
   a. **Conidia production**

10. Tease preparation reveals a mold with septate hyphae. Which of the following might be seen in a slide culture of this organism?
    c. **Macroconidia**

CHAPTER 36
Dermatophytes and Other Agents of Superficial Mycoses

Suggested Answers to

A 16-year-old man presented to his physician with an itchy, scaly, red rash on his hands. He had been spending his summer vacation participating on a swimming team at the YMCA. Physical examination revealed some cracks and fissures in the skin between the fourth and fifth toes of both feet. There was some inflammation and scaling of the skin adjacent to the fifth toe on the left foot. Except for the hands, no additional skin rash was detected. KOH preparation of the lesions on the foot revealed fungal hyphae. However, repeated KOH preparation of the rash from the hands revealed no hyphae at all.

Questions:

1. What is your diagnosis? **The patient has tinea pedis (athlete's foot) and has developed the "id reaction" on his hands.**

2. Why was the KOH preparation from the hands negative? **The KOH preparation from the hands is negative because the "id reaction" is an allergic reaction associated with a dermatophyte infection located elsewhere in** the body. When the primary infection is treated, the "id reaction" also resolves. The term "id" is short for dermatophytid.

3. What are some of the organisms likely to be involved? **Some common organisms associated with tinea pedis include *Trichophyton mentagrophytes, Trichophyton rubrum,* and *Epidermophyton floccosum.***

Answers to

Review Questions

1. A patient presents with a chronic infection of the fingernails. Which of the following organisms is the most likely cause?
   b. *Trichophyton rubrum*

2. A culture of skin scrapings reveals a fungus that produces club-shaped macroconidia and no microconidia. Which of the following organisms is most likely?
   a. *Epidermophyton floccosum*

3. *Trichophyton mentagrophytes* can be distinguished from *Trichophyton rubrum* by which of the following?
   d. **All of the above**

4. The most common cause of tinea capitis in the United States today is:
   d. *Trichophyton tonsurans.*

5. Which of the following are characteristic of dermatophytes?
   b. **"Spaghetti and meatballs"**

6. Addition of which of the following to the culture media will aid in the identification of the species of *Trichophyton?*

    d.   **Thiamine**

7. *Epidermophyton floccosum* is associated with which of the following?

    d.   **none of the above**

8. Which of the following causes tinea cruris (jock itch)?

    b.   ***Epidermophyton floccosum***

9. Which of the following organisms is most likely to be transmitted by contact with animals?

    d.   ***Microsporum canis***

10. Use of polished rice grains or rice grain medium will aid in the identification of which of the following?

    c.   ***Microsporum audouinii***

CHAPTER 37
Agents of Subcutaneous Mycoses

Suggested Answers to

A 54-year-old woman presented to her physician because of a nonhealing wound on her finger. The patient stated that she had developed a painful swollen index finger several weeks before. Eventually the wound broke down and formed an ulcer that would not heal. Recently she had developed some red, painful streaks along her forearm and a swollen nodule over her elbow. The patient was an executive with a major computer software corporation. In her leisure time she was an avid rose gardener and had won several prizes for her roses.

Questions:

1. What disease does the patient have? What is the causative organism? **Sporotrichosis. *Sporothrix schenkii* is the causative organism. The description of the infection in this patient is classic. The organism is found in decaying vegetation, especially sphagnum moss, favored by gardeners. Sporotrichosis is especially associated with rose gardeners, because the organism can be introduced into the skin by the sharp thorns.**

2. If you wish to demonstrate the organism in a direct preparation from the finger wound, how would you process the specimen? What would you expect to see? **In infected tissue, *Sporothrix schenkii* is a small yeast that is nearly impossible to identify in KOH prep. It requires special fungal stains to recognize it in microscopic preparations. Because the yeast is quite small and has a highly variable appearance, it can be confused with tissue debris in standard fungal stains. Therefore, it may be necessary to digest the tissue with salivary gland diastase prior to applying the fungal stains.**

3. How would you confirm the identity of the organism in culture? ***Sporothrix schenkii* is dimorphic. It is quite easy to culture on standard fungal media. At room temperature it grows as a mold that produces conidia. The delicate conidia are produced on top of conidiophores, like petals on the head of a flower. Larger conidia can also be produced directly from the hyphae. Confirmation of thermal dimorphism is achieved by culturing the mold on rich agar, such as BHI blood agar, at 37°C. This yields moist, creamy colonies containing the characteristic yeast cells.**

Answers to

Review Questions

1. A patient presents with chromoblastomycosis. A sample of the infected material is sent to the laboratory for direct examination by KOH prep. Which of the following would you expect to see?

   b. Pigmented sclerotic bodies

2. Which of the following organisms causes chromoblastomycosis?

   d. All of the above

3. A patient presents with mycotic mycetoma of the foot. Small granules are recovered from pus draining from the infection. What are these granules composed of?

   a. Masses of hyphae

4. Which of the following organisms is dimorphic?

   c. *Sporothrix schenkii*

5. Growth in culture at 42°C will help distinguish which of the following organisms?

   d. *Wangiella dermatitidis* from *Exophiala jeanselmei*

6. *Pseudoallescheria boydii* produces which of the following type(s) of conidia production?

   d. none of the above

7. *Exophiala jeanselmei* may cause mycotic mycetoma of the extremities. What color granules will it produce?

   c. Black

8. Which of the following organisms is most likely to produce sexual spores in culture?

   b. *Pseudoallescheria boydii*

9. Which of the following organisms is dematiaceous?

   d. All of the above

10. Which of the following organisms produces vase-shaped phialides?

    a. *Phialophora verrucosa*

CHAPTER 38
Systemic Dimorphic Fungi

Suggested Answers to

A 45-year-old male patient developed a flulike respiratory infection. He worked in a cotton textile mill in eastern North Carolina, and had never been outside of the state of North Carolina in his life. His job in the mill was to receive and open the bales of cotton that had been shipped in from other parts of the United States including Arizona.

The flulike illness became progressively severe, and the patient developed signs of high fever and pneumonia. He was admitted to the hospital, but died within a few days, before a definitive diagnosis could be made.

An autopsy was performed, which revealed infection involving many organs of the body, including lungs, liver, lymph nodes, spleen, kidneys, and adrenal glands. Sections of the involved tissues revealed large spherules as shown in Figure 38-17. Within a week culture grew a white mold that produced arthroconidia.

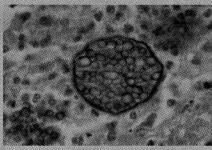

FIGURE 38-17 Photomicrograph of structures found in tissue of patient.

Questions:

1. What is the name of the organism that caused the infection? What is the disease called? **Organism: *Coccidioides immitis*. Disease: Coccidioidomycosis (disseminated).**

2. What is the relationship of the white mold grown in culture to the spherule seen in tissue sections? ***Coccidioides immitis* is dimorphic. The parasitic phase found in tissue is the spherule containing endospores. The saprophytic phase found in nature is a mold that produces arthroconidia. Since fungal cultures are incubated at room temperature, cultures will yield the mold phase of the organism. The exoantigen immunodiffusion test can be used to prove that the mold is *C. immitis*. Conversion of the mold to the spherule phase is extremely difficult and beyond the ability of most hospital laboratories. Always remember to use extreme caution when handling *Coccidioides immitis* in the laboratory, since the arthroconidia are highly infectious. The organism should always be kept in a biological safety hood. Screw-top tube media, not Petri dishes, should be used.**

3. Because the patient had never traveled outside the state of North Carolina, how did he contract the infection? ***Coccidioides immitis* has a very restricted geographical distribution; it is found in the desert southwest in the United States. However, in this case, the cotton bales that it was his job to receive and open came from Arizona. It is very likely this cotton was contaminated with arthroconidia from the Arizona soil. As he opened the cotton bales, the arthroconidia became airborne, and he inhaled them into his lungs.**

4. Is the type of clinical infection this patient had typical of most infections caused by this organism? **Most people who develop coccidioidomycosis have an inapparent infection or a flu-like illness ("valley fever"). Fewer than one percent of patients develop the kind of devastating disseminated infection that this patient did. Immunocompromised patients are more prone to disseminated infections, but in some cases the reason for dissemination is not apparent.**

Answers to

Review Questions

1. Which of the following characteristics is NOT generally associated with the systemic true pathogenic fungi?
   d.   **Normal flora in humans**

2. Which of the following is (are) characteristic of *Histoplasma capsulatum?*
   d.   **All of the above**

3. Which of the following organisms produces arthroconidia?
   a.   ***Coccidioides immitis***

4. Which of the following is characteristic of the yeast phase of *Histoplasma capsulatum?*
   d.   **None of the above**

5. A sample of infected skin from a patient with cutaneous blastomycosis is submitted to the laboratory and examined directly under the microscope. Which of the following is likely to be seen?
   a.   **Large yeast with single broad-based bud**

6. Which of the following tests are useful in identifying *Histoplasma capsulatum* in culture?
   d.   **All of the above**

7. Which of the following cities is found in an area endemic for histoplasmosis?
   c.   **Nashville, Tennessee**

8. Which of the following is considered to be the most infectious agent?
   b.   **Arthroconidia of *Coccidioides immitis***

9. KOH preparation from an ulcer in the mouth reveals a large yeast surrounded by small radial buds. What is the identity of the organism?
   a.   ***Paracoccidioides brasiliensis***

10. Biopsy of an ulcer in the mouth reveals yeast forms characteristic of *Histoplasma capsulatum*. Which of the following statements concerning this patient's infection is true?
    b.   **The organism spread to the mouth from the lungs.**

CHAPTER 39
Opportunistic Fungi

Suggested Answers to

A 62-year-old male patient had a 15-year history of autoimmune hemolytic anemia. He had been treated with corticosteroid drugs and had responded well. However, when the steroids were stopped, the anemia recurred. Steroids were reinstituted and he was also treated with immunosuppressive and cytotoxic drugs. Approximately 1 month later he presented with a swollen abdomen, fever, and severe headache. He was noted to have an unstable gait. Some fluid was removed from the abdominal cavity by needle and syringe. This fluid was thick, viscous, and very mucoid. A spinal tap revealed elevated cerebrospinal fluid pressure. The fluid had a low glucose value and elevated protein. Lymphocytes were moderately increased, but there were no neutrophils.

Questions

1. What diagnosis do you suspect? Why? **Cryptococcosis. The patient is at high risk for opportunistic fungal infection because of corticosteroid, immunosuppressive, and cytotoxic drug therapy. *Cryptococcus neoformans* is an opportunistic organism that is very commonly associated with meningitis, but with relatively few lymphocytes and no neutrophils in the spinal fluid. These findings are typical of cryptococcal meningitis rather than meningitis caused by bacteria or even other fungi. Supportive evidence includes the character of the abdominal fluid, which was viscous and mucoid. *Cryptococcus neoformans* possesses a mucoid capsule, which may be responsible for the lack of a prominent cell response to the organism in the spinal fluid or the abdominal fluid.**

2. What is the most rapid test you could perform to confirm this diagnosis? What other tests might be helpful? **The most rapid diagnostic test would be to perform an India ink prep on the spinal fluid and the abdominal fluid. A positive India ink prep would reveal the capsule of *C. neoformans,* which would provide a definitive diagnosis, since no other organisms possess such a capsule. Only approximately 50% of patients with cryptococcal meningitis have a positive India ink prep with spinal fluid due to the low number of organisms. The mucoid character of the abdominal fluid leads one to suspect that there are a large number of organisms in that fluid, and that an India ink prep of the abdominal fluid is very likely to be positive. Detection of cryptococcal antigen in spinal fluid and abdominal fluid would also be diagnostic but the test takes longer to perform. Of course, the specimen should also be cultured. The mucoid capsule could also be demonstrated in smear preparations of the abdominal fluid by alcian blue or mucicarmine stains, which are specific for acid mucopolysaccharides.**

3. Do you expect other organ systems to be involved in this case? Why? **It is very likely that this patient has involvement of other organ systems in the body. The portal of entry for *Cryptococcus neoformans* is the respiratory tract. From there it may spread to other parts of the body, with meningitis being the most common form of disseminated infection. The meningitis may occur without involvement of other organs; however, the presence of organisms in large numbers in abdominal fluid suggests widespread involvement of abdominal organs, especially the intestinal tract. In such cases, the organism probably has gained access to the blood stream, and it is likely that many other organs have been seeded by the organism. Blood and bone marrow cultures are very likely to yield *Cryptococcus neoformans.* Involvement of the kidneys could be detected by urine cultures.**

Answers to

Review Questions

1. Which of the following provides definitive evidence that the patient has an opportunistic infection of the lung?
   d. **None of the above**

2. KOH prep of sinus tissue reveals broad, non-septate fungal hyphae. Which of the following organisms is most likely present?
   d. ***Rhizopus* species**

3. Which of the following provides the most definitive evidence that a patient has pulmonary aspergillosis?
   d. **Presence of fungal hyphae in sputum smear and *Aspergillus fumigatus* in sputum culture**

4. A yeast is recovered from a sputum culture. Which of the following would provide definitive evidence that the yeast is *Cryptococcus neoformans?*
   b. **Positive alcian blue stain**

5. Which of the following organisms is dimorphic?
   a. ***Penicillium marneffei***

6. Which of the following organisms is part of the normal flora of the mouth and intestinal tract of humans?
   c. ***Candida albicans***

7. Observation of yeast with pseudohyphae is presumptive evidence of which of the following?
   a. ***Candida albicans***

8. Which of the following predispose to an opportunistic infection?
   d. **All of the above**

9. Which of the following is presumptive evidence that an observed organism is *Aspergillus* species?
   b. **Calcium oxalate crystals**

10. Which of the following tests can distinguish meningitis caused by *Cryptococcus neoformans* from meningitis caused by *Candida albicans?*
    a. **India ink prep of spinal fluid**

CHAPTER 40

Saprobic Fungi Encountered in Clinical Specimens

Suggested Answers to

CASE STUDY

A 25-year-old male patient underwent endoscopic sinus surgery for chronic, recurrent episodes of sinusitis. He also had a history of food allergies in childhood and seasonal allergic rhinitis (hay fever). Microscopic examination of the sinus tissue revealed numerous eosinophils and impacted mucus. Culture of the sinus tissue revealed well developed fuzzy dark brown mold colonies in 4 days. Colony reverse was black. Curved macroconidia with transverse septa were produced from conidiophores.

Questions:

1. What is the name of the organism cultured? **Curvularia species.**

2. What is the significance of the organism in this case? **Although *Curvularia* species most commonly is an environmental contaminant in cultures, it has also been associated with allergic sinusitis. In this case, it is very likely the cause of the patient's chronic sinusitis.**

The culture should not be discarded as contaminated.

3. What other organisms might also have been expected in this culture? **Other organisms associated with allergic sinusitis include the dematiaceous fungi *Bipolaris* species, *Cladosporium* species, and *Alternaria* species, as well as *Aspergillus* species and some of the Zygomycetes.**

Answers to

Review Questions

1. Which of the following is (are) not characteristic of Zygomycetes?
   c. **Vesicle**

2. Which of the following organisms is dimorphic?
   a. ***Penicillium marneffei***

3. Which of the following organisms produce macroconidia?
   d. **All of the above**

4. Which of the following organisms possess dematiaceous, septate hyphae?
   a. ***Bipolaris* species**

5. Which of the following is NOT characteristic of *Penicillium* species?
   c. **Tuberculate macroconidia**

6. Which of the saprophytic fungi may be confused with a dimorphic pathogen?
   b. ***Chrysosporium* species**

7. Which of the following organisms produce rhizoids?
   b. *Absidia* species

8. Which of the following organisms produces a vesicle?
   d. **All of the above**

9. Blue-green colonies are commonly observed with which of the following organisms?
   d. **None of the above**

10. Which of the following are most likely to be confused with *Aspergillus* species microscopically?
    a. *Syncephalastrum* species

CHAPTER 41
Yeasts

Suggested Answers to

CASE STUDY

A culture is requested on a portion of a heart valve allograft that has been replaced in surgery. The tissue is minced and placed on blood agar and chocolate agar and in thioglycollate broth. After 24 hours incubation at 37°C, the thioglycollate appears cloudy and both the blood agar and chocolate agar show moderate growth of white, glossy colonies that are catalase positive. The direct Gram stain reveals a few large oval cells with a single bud.

Questions:

1. What test should be done on this isolate to confirm that a yeast is present? **A direct wet prep should be done to determine if the colonies are yeasts.**

2. What test should be done on this isolate to rule out *Candida albicans*? *Cryptococcus neoformans*? **A germ tube test will help to rule out *Candida albicans*. Most *Candida albicans* isolates are germ tube positive. An India ink test will rule out *Cryptococcus neoformans*.**

Cryptococcus neoformans **has a distinct capsule, but** *Candida albicans* **does not.**

3. If the isolate is *Candida albicans*, what would you expect to see microscopically on cornmeal agar? *Candida albicans* **forms pseudohyphae, clusters of blastoconidia at the constrictions of the pseudohyphae, and thick-walled, terminal chlamydospores on cornmeal agar.**

Answers to

Review Questions

1. A yeast isolate is germ tube positive and sucrose positive. On cornmeal agar pseudohyphae, clusters of blastoconidia and terminal chlamydospores are seen. The organism may be identified as:
   b. *Candida albicans.*

2. Speciation of *Candida* (other than *albicans*) requires results of which tests?
   d. **Sugar assimilations**

3. A presumptive identification of *Cryptococcus* in a case of meningitis can be reported if the following is/are seen:
   c. **encapsulated yeast cells in India ink prep of CSF.**

4. Which of the following species produce germ tubes?
   b. *Candida albicans*

5. Which of the following tests can differentiate *Candida albicans* from *Candida krusei*?
   a. **Sucrose assimilation**

6. A yeast forms long blastoconidia that tend to form parallel lines with the pseudohyphae, giving the appearance of "logs in a steam." It does not assimilate maltose or melibiose. What is the identity of this organism?
   c. ***Candida keyfur***

7. A yeast colony with a red pigment is isolated. What is the most likely identity of this isolate?
   d. ***Rhodotorula rubra***

8. Which of the following forms arthroconidia on cornmeal agar?
   a. ***Geotrichum candidum***

9. A test that will differentiate *Cryptococcus neoformans* from other *Cryptococcus* species is:
   d. **Niger seed agar.**

10. Which of the following conditions or treatments predisposes patients to yeast infections?
    d. **All of the above**

CHAPTER 42
Basic Concepts and Techniques in Parasitology

Answers to

Review Questions

1. Which of the following are metazoans?
   d. Both a and b are metazoans.

2. Which of the following best defines "reservoir host"?
   c. An organism that harbors the same stage of the parasite that is found in humans.

3. How do parasitic organisms overcome the difficulties they face in transmitting the next generation to a suitable host?
   b. Parasitic organisms have a greater reproductive potential than do most free-living species thus increasing the chances of transfer to a suitable host.

4. Which of the following are necessary for the transmission of parasitic disease to occur?
   d. All of the above are necessary for the transmission of parasitic disease.

5. A stool sample is collected from a patient suspected of infection with *Entamoeba histolytica*. The stool sample is liquid. What stage of the life cycle of *Entamoeba* is most likely to be observed in the specimen?
   b. The trophozoite

6. Individuals infected with *Taenia* species may undergo an increased parasitic burden by which of the following?
   c. Budding of the cysticercus

7. Monecious helminths are able to:
   d. Only a and b are true.

8. Eggs of *Paragonimus westermani* are only able to develop into metacercariae if they:
   c. are deposited into an aquatic environment with the appropriate species of snail.

9. *Giardia lamblia* is able to resist the host's defenses by:
   a. changing surface antigens.

10. Direct wet films of fecal samples are examined to detect:
    a. protozoan cysts and helminth eggs.

CHAPTER 43

Specimen Collection and Processing for Parasite Examinations

Suggested Answers to

CASE STUDY

A 3-year-old girl was referred for evaluation of diarrhea. One month prior, the patient had been having chronic abdominal pain and gas to frank diarrhea for the preceding 1 to 2 weeks. On the morning of her evaluation, the patient's diarrhea was yellow, foul-smelling, and frothy. Specimen was collected for culture and ova and parasite examination. After 48 hours, the stool culture was reported as negative for enteric pathogens and the ova and parasite examination was positive for pear-shaped trophozoites 12 to 15 μm long with two bilateral nuclei.

Questions:

1. Which parasite was found in the stool specimen? **The trophozoites were those of the flagellate protozoan *Giardia lamblia*.**

2. How is this parasite transmitted? **Ingestion of the cysts is required for the initiation of infection. In children in day-care settings or orphanages, the cysts are often transmitted directly from person to person.**

3. How can infection with this organism be prevented? **To prevent direct person-to-person spread, good hygiene practice (handwashing) is highly recommended.**

Answers to

Review Questions

1. Parasites that may be found in sputum specimens include:
   d. ***Paragonimus westermani* and hookworm.**

2. The trophozoite stage of a parasite can be recovered from a soft fecal specimen submitted for parasitic examination if the specimen:
   d. **is placed into PVA solution 30 minutes after defecation.**

3. In cases of suspected infection with *Enterobius vermicularis,* the preferred specimen is:
   c. **cellulose acetate.**

4. *Schistosoma haematobium* is best detected by examination of:
   a. **urine sediment**.

5. When stool examination is negative, the preferred specimen for the diagnosis of paragonimiasis is:
   c. **expectorated sputum.**

6. *Enterobius vermicularis* infection is usually diagnosed by:
   d. **finding eggs in perianal specimens.**

7. In which specimen is the eggs of *Schistosoma haematobium* most likely to be found?
   c. **Urine**

8. Immunocompromised hosts have been found to have an increased susceptibility to:

   e. all of the above

9. Knowledge of its nocturnal periodicity is especially important in the diagnosis of:

   c. *Wuchereria bancrofti.*

10. Hematuria is a typical sign of human infection caused by:

   c. *Schistosoma haematobium.*

CHAPTER 44
Intestinal and Atrial Protozoans

Suggested Answers to

A 46-year-old male patient is admitted to the hospital with severe dysentery, fever, and hepatomegaly. Trophozoites with thin pseudopodia and a single nucleus having a distinct, central endosome are recovered from a liver biopsy. Although no cysts are detected in a fecal specimen collected from the patient, some trophozoites are identified. The genus and species of the infecting protozoan is most likely:

Questions:

1. a. Endolimax nana
    b. Chilomastix mesnili
    c. Isospora belli
    d. **Entamoeba histolytica**
    e. Blastocystis hominis

2. Cysts of the protozoan in question number 1 could have which of the following characteristics?
    a. Chromatodial bodies
    b. Two nuclei
    c. Four nuclei
    d. **All of the above**

3. What staining technique would be most appropriate to identify the trophozoites and cysts of the protozoan in question number 1?
    a. Giemsa staining
    b. **Trichrome staining**
    c. Modified acid-fast staining
    d. Gram staining

Answers to

Review Questions

1. One possible result of giardiasis is malabsorption syndrome. It is most likely due to which of the following?
    d. **Damage to the intestinal lining caused by *Giardia's* sucking disk**

2. While residing in the human intestine *Giardia lamblia* relies on _____ for nutrition.
    a. **the contents of the intestine and occasional ingestion of host epithelial cells**

3. Which of the following protozoans have a cytosome and a short flagellum that resembles a shepherd's crook?
    a. ***Chilomastix mesnili***

4. What role to micronuclei play in the life cycle of *Balantidium coli?*
    b. **They are exchanged during conjugation.**

5. Persons with which of the following occupations would be most likely to become infected with *Balantidium coli?*
    b. **Pork ranchers**

6. Which of the following is least likely to be found in a fecal specimen?

   d. ***Entamoeba gingivalis***

7. Why are asymptomatic individuals who are infected with *Giardia lamblia* more important in the epidemiology of giardiasis than are symptomatic individuals who are experiencing severe diarrhea?

   d. Because symptomatic individuals pass the infectious cyst stage in their feces

8. *Trichomonas hominis* can be distinguished from *Trichomonas vaginalis* based on:

   d. Only a and b are true.

9. A 24-year-old woman seeks medical attention for what she believes is a severe yeast infection after an over-the-counter yeast medication fails to work. The symptoms that she is experiencing include a profuse, foul-smelling, whitish, vaginal discharge and bright red spots on the vaginal mucosa. She also reported severe itching of the vaginal mucosa and burning on urination. Which of the following is identified in a vaginal smear of the patient?

   b. A teardrop-shaped trophozoite with an undulating membrane that begins at the anterior end of the cell and extends about half the length of the cell

10. The physician might prescribe which of the following to treat the young woman in question #9?

    a. Metronidazole

CHAPTER 45

Plasmodia and Other Blood and Tissue Protozoans

Suggested Answers to

Questions:

1. What staining technique(s) would be appropriate for the peripheral blood smear taken from the patient? **Giemsa or Wright stain.**

2. How is malaria transmitted to humans? **By the bite of an infected *Anopheles* mosquito.**

3. List the four species of *Plasmodium* that cause malaria in humans. ***Plasmodium vivax, malariae, P. falciparum, P. ovale.***

Questions:

1. What gender of *Anopheles* mosquito transmits *Plasmodium* to humans? **The female mosquito.**

2. During what time(s) of day are mosquito bites most common? **Evening.**

3. What actions could be taken to help prevent the transmission of malaria? **Use insect repellents, sleep indoors with screens over the windows.**

4. Why is proximity to water significant to the transmission of malaria? **The mosquitos lay their eggs in the water and the larva develop there.**

Suggested Answers to

CASE STUDY 3

A 30-year-old homosexual man was well until January 1981 when he developed esophageal and oral candidiasis. He was treated with amphotericin B, which resolved the infection. The man was hospitalized in February 1981 for *Pneumocystis* pneumonia and was successfully treated with trimethoprim-sulfamethoxazole (TMP/SMX). The esophageal candidiasis recurred after the pneumonia was diagnosed and an esophageal biopsy revealed that he also had cytomegalovirus (CMV).

(Note: This case study was one of the first cases of pneumocystis pneumonia that led to the identification of HIV. It was reprinted by CDC as a part of their 50th year anniversary.)

Questions:

1. What can you conclude about the overall health of the patient? **The patient is severely immunocompromised.**

2. What is the most probable source of the candidiasis? **The patient's normal flora.**

Answers to

Review Questions

Use the following case study for questions 1–3.

An optometrist sees a 17-year-old contact lens wearing male patient who complains of chronic irritation of his left eye. On examination, the optometrist does not see anything unusual, and recommends that the patient not wear his contacts for 1 week. She reschedules a return visit for the patient in 1 week.

Four days later the patient calls to tell the doctor that the eye has not improved and is now extremely painful. The optometrist refers the patient to an ophthalmologist. After questioning the patient, the optometrist learned that the patient prepares his own saline solution and uses a cold disinfection method.

1. Based on the information that is provided what would be your tentative diagnosis?
    d. *Acanthamoeba* **keratitis**

2. If your tentative diagnosis is correct, what test(s) would you order to confirm your suspicions?
    c. **Take a corneal scraping to stain and examine for the presence of trophozoites and cysts.**

3. Assuming that a corneal abrasion is not the cause of the problem, what life style stages are possible in the infectious agent?
    b. **A trophozoite and a cyst**

Questions 4–8. Choose the correct response for each of the possible pathogens.

4. *Toxoplasma gondii:*
    d. **Oocysts, a congenital infection of the CNS of a fetus**

5. *Plasmodium:*
    a. **Black water fever,** *Anopheles* **mosquito**

6. *Naegleria fowleri:*
    d. **A hot tub, a disease that is usually diagnosed at autopsy**

7. *Trypanosoma* species:
    b. **Crithidial form of the disease, epimastigote stage of the parasite**

8. *Babesia* species:
    c. **An individual who has had a splenectomy,** *Ixoides* **ticks**

Use the following information for questions 9 and 10.

After being bitten by an infected arthropod, the patient experiences a high fever, night sweats, and joint and muscle pain. The chronic form of the disease develops in about 9 months.

9. The causative agent is:
    d. *Trypanosoma.*

10. What life cycle stages of the parasite could be observed in the patient's blood?
    d. **Both a and c**

CHAPTER 46
Intestinal Helminths

Suggested Answers to

CASE STUDY

A 49-year-old man, a recent Russian immigrant, is admitted to the hospital for a possible intestinal blockage. When taking the patient's history, the physician learned that the patient has been experiencing chronic diarrhea, flatulence, and abdominal cramps. Further questioning revealed that the consumption of pickled fish, usually pike, was common in the patient's home village. Cestode eggs but no proglottids were recovered from the patient's feces. Based on this information answer the following questions.

Questions:

1. What genus and species of cestode is the most likely culprit? *Diphyllobothrium latum.*

2. Why were no proglottids recovered from the patient's fecal sample? *D. latum releases its eggs from a uterine pore rather than in proglottids that break off of the end of the tapeworm.*

3. How could the infection have been avoided? **By completely cooking the fish, rather than pickling it, which does not kill the eggs.**

4. What treatment is recommended for treatment of infections with this cestode? *Praziquantal or niclosimide.*

Answers to

Review Questions

1. Nematodes that parasitize humans spend:
   d. Both b and c are true.

2. A 3-year-old boy is examined in an outpatient clinic for itching and bleeding of the perianal skin. His mother observed a small, round worm protruding from his anus but did not have the presence of mind to bring the worm to the doctor. Which of the following did the doctor most likely give the mother for use on the child to aid in diagnosis? Which drug is likely to have been prescribed?
   d. A small paddle covered with sticky tape, mebendazole

3. A 47-year-old female Korean immigrant presents with chronic indigestion and mild jaundice. The physician determines that sushi dishes are a favorite of the patient. While in Korea, the patient worked as a fisherwoman. What is the likely diagnosis and treatment?
   a. *Clonorchis sinesis*, praziquantel

4. A patient is infected with *Necator americanus*. How did the infection probably occur?
   d. By walking barefooted on contaminated soil

5. Infection with which of the following parasites is most likely to result in the development of serious symptoms?
   d. *Taenia solium* cysticerci

6. Human infection with _____ may occur on ingestion of infected grain or grain products.

   b. *Hymenolepsis diminuta*

7. A resident specializing in tropical medicine examines a 7-year-old girl. She is obviously small for her age and is anemic. The child has experienced alternating bouts of diarrhea and dysentery for at least 6 months. A fecal examination reveals football-shaped eggs with polar plugs at both ends. How was the child most likely infected?

   d. **By playing in contaminated soil**

8. What drug is prescribed to the child in question 7?

   c. **Mebendazole**

9. A difference between *Diphyllobothrium latum* and many other tapeworms is:

   d. **that its eggs are released through a uterine pore rather than in proglottids.**

10. How are infections with *Necator americanus* and *Ancylostoma duodenale* differentiated?

   d. **None of the above**

CHAPTER 47
Blood and Tissue Helminths

Suggested Answers to

CASE STUDY 1

(Adapted from Lucey & Maguire, 1993).

During a trip to Kenya, six American students became ill with diarrhea and fever several weeks after swimming in a slow-moving stream in the Machakos district. All were treated at a hospital in Nairobi where a diagnosis of malaria was considered. One student, a 21-year-old man, developed fever, sweats, and abdominal pain 4 weeks after swimming in the stream. He continued to feel unwell, and 2 weeks later he developed more fever, sweats, chills, and mild nonbloody diarrhea. He received a 4-day course of chloroquine. His symptoms improved, but he developed dull pain in the lumbar region and numbness in his toes. He subsequently became unable to void and he became so weak in his legs that he could not walk. On examination he was unable to lift his legs and had diminished sensation and absent deep tendon reflexes in the legs. The white blood cell (WBC) count was 9,600 with 33% neutrophils and 47% eosinophils. The cerebrospinal fluid WBC count was 44/mm^3, the red blood cell count was 36/mm^3, and the protein was 84 mg/100 mL. A computed tomography myelogram of the spine showed diffuse enlargement of the lower thoracic spinal cord.

Questions

1. Name three pathogens or diseases that could cause the above symptoms. **Malaria, schistosomiasis, hepatitis.**

2. Based on the contents of this chapter what is the most likely causative parasite? **Schistosomiasis.**

3. What clinical samples would you collect and what diagnostic tests would you request? **Feces, urine, biopsy.**

Suggested Answers to

CASE STUDY 2

An 8-year-old white boy was admitted to a hospital with fever of unknown origin and nasal catarrh of 1 week duration. During infancy the child had no major illnesses. On numerous occasions, he had been observed eating dirt in the yard. The family had no house pets. On first admission the child was pale, with a temperature of 101°F and a slightly enlarged spleen. His hemoglobin was 7.2% gm, WBC count was 32,000/mm³, with 64% eosinophils. Radiographs of the chest showed streaky, abnormal shadows in the right upper and both lower lobes. A tentative diagnosis was made of iron deficiency anemia and possible visceral larva migrans. He was treated with ferrous sulfate and ampicillin and released. Three weeks later the child was readmitted in a semicomatose state with a 10-day history of shaking spells and ataxia. The WBC count was 9,100/mm³ with 4% eosinophils. Cerebrospinal fluid sugar was 88 mg % and protein 320 mg %. An electroencephalogram was abnormal, but a burr-hole exploration and left carotid angiograph were normal. Convulsions were poorly controlled by antiepileptic agents and the patient died 3 weeks after his second admission and 7 weeks following his first admission.

On autopsy granulomata in various stages of development were found in the liver, heart, and brain. The lungs were edematous and there were numerous granulomata containing infiltrates of eosinophils, neutrophils, lymphocytes, and plasma cells. These were considered to be more chronic lesions. In contrast, the numerous granulomata in the gray and white matter of the cerebral hemispheres, cerebellum, and brain stem appeared to be of more recent origin than those in the visceral organs.

Questions:

1. Based on your knowledge of this chapter, what is the most likely causative agent? **Trichinella spiralis.**

2. Explain the reasons for the severity of the clinical symptoms. **Because of dissemination of the organism throughout the patient's body and encystment of the parasite in various muscles including the heart, the patient probably reinfected himself (when eating dirt) several times.**

Answers to

Review Questions

1. You are the microbiologist at a large metropolitan hospital. A patient, who has recently arrived from Africa, is admitted to the hospital and has numerous nonspecific symptoms but also has what the resident-physician describes as Calabar swelling. The astute resident suspects the patient has loiasis but informs you that the patient, due to his religious beliefs, will agree to only one blood sample. It is now 10 PM; you should advise the physician to:
   c. **try to convince the patient that several blood samples must be taken.**

2. A man from Brazil is admitted to the hospital with portal hypertension, polyps in the large intestine, and splenomegaly. What is the likely causative agent?
   b. *Schistosoma mansoni*

3. You are a cercaria of *S. haematobium*. After secretly entering your favorite human where will you first go to mature?
   d. **The venous plexuses of the pelvis**

4. Another name for river blindness is:
   b. **Sowda**

5. You are an epidemiologist working for the WHO in charge of investigating cystic hydatid disease in Spain. Your most effective advice to the local authorities to help prevent the spread of this disease to humans would include: (1) to increase the chlorine content of the local drinking water; (2) thoroughly educate the public on personal hygiene measures; (3) to stop the feeding of animal organs to other domestic animals; (4) to trap and sample wild carnivores for disease. Then, to recommend extensive hunting of carnivores if they carry the disease. Pick one pair of answers below.

   b. 3, 4

6. The most commonly used diagnostic tests for active trichinosis infections include: (1) biopsy; (2) complement fixation; (3) polymerase chain reaction; (4) antibody detection. Pick one pair of the answers below.

   a. 1, 2

7. (True or False) The definitive diagnosis of filarial infections is complicated by antigenic cross-reactivity between genera/species and the duration of the host's antibody response. This cross-reactivity would be negated by the use of the following assays:

   a. True
   b. True
   c. False
   d. False

8. Based on your understanding of epidemiology and the host range of the parasites listed below, which is the parasite most likely to be eradicated by a concerted effort of the WHO?

   c. *Dracunculus medinensis*

9. Which of the following parasites are commonly associated with domestic dogs: (1) *Toxocara canis;* (2) *Dirofilaria* species; (3) *Ancylostoma caninum.* (4) *Echinococcus granulosus.*

   d. 1, 2, 3, 4

10. For the geographic area in which the disease is most prevalent, match the parasite with its most likely vector/intermediate host. Use each answer only once.

   a. ***Schistosoma mansoni***   4. **Snail.**

   b. ***Onchocerca volvulus***   5. ***Simulium*** **(black fly).**

   c. ***Wuchereria bancrofti***   3. ***Culex*** **and** ***Anopheles*** **mosquitos.**

   d. ***Dirofilaria species***   6. ***Aedes*** **mosquito.**

   e. ***Loa loa***   1. ***Chrysops*** **fly.**

   f. ***Dracunculus medinensis***   2. **Copepod.**

CHAPTER 48

Basic Concepts and Techniques in Virology

Suggested Answers to

An 18-year-old woman, with a sore throat, presented at the college health care facility. She had been well until 3 days ago, when she experienced the gradual onset of malaise, anorexia, and mild sore throat. The symptoms had intensified, and she now felt that her throat was "on fire." She presented as feverish, with a frontal headache, and had lost complete interest in food and cigarettes. She had received the DPT vaccine as a child. Her physical exam showed T 39°C, BP 126/70, P 92, R 18. The patient appeared acutely ill. Her skin showed no rash or jaundice; her throat was intensely red and swollen, with a yellowish exudate on the left tonsil. There was several tender, enlarged lymph nodes, with no signs of meningeal irritation. Chest, heart, abdomen, and neurologic exams were normal. Blood analysis showed a hematocrit of 39%, white cell (WBC) count 14,000, and differential of 52% polymorphonuclear cells (PMNs), 45% lymphocytes, 3% monocytes, and platelets 100,000. Urine and chest x-rays were normal. The following day, the throat culture showed α-hemolytic streptococci and the Monospot was negative. Transaminases were elevated to twice normal levels. WBC, 16,000; differential: 48% PMNs, 50% lymphs (3% are atypical), 2% monos. The patient was treated with aspirin and warm, saltwater gargles. Her throat remained sore for the next 2 days. The following day, her temperature dropped to 38°C and she began to feel somewhat better. The Monospot test was positive by this time.

Questions:

1. What is your differential diagnosis and what laboratory tests should be ordered to make a microbiologic diagnosis? **The clinical picture is typical of infectious mononucleosis caused by Epstein-Barr virus (EBV). Other viruses (herpes simplex, coxsackieviruses, and adenoviruses) can also cause pharyngitis, as do certain bacteria (*Streptococcus pyogenes* and *Neisseria gonorrhoeae*). Cytomegalovirus may cause a mononucleosis condition, but without the sore throat. Diphtheria is unlikely, since the patient was immunized. Immediate laboratory tests should include throat culture for *S. pyogenes* and a heterophile test (monospot test).**

2. In view of these laboratory findings, what would be your diagnostic impression? **Streptococcal pharyngitis can be ruled out, since only α-hemolytic colonies were found on cul-** ture. **The heterophile test can be negative in early infectious mononucleosis. The liver function tests and the finding of several atypical lymphocytes support the diagnosis of infectious mononucleosis.**

3. What was this infection and how is this infection transmitted? **This is a typical case of infectious mononucleosis, with the chief findings of fever, pharyngitis, lymphocytosis with atypical cells, and a positive heterophile test. The last two features can appear several days after the patient presents. EBV is present in saliva, and transmission between young adults is primarily by kissing. EBV infects oropharyngeal cells, causing the pharyngitis. Over 90% of the adults in the United States have antibodies to this virus.**

Answers to

Review Questions

1. The viral structure consisting of the genome and protein coat is called a(n):
   d.   nucleocapsid.

2. Acyclovir inhibits herpes simplex viruses. To do so, it interferes with:
   b.   viral nucleic acid metabolism.

3. Interferons inhibit viral growth by primarily affecting:
   b.   host protein synthesis.

4. Which viral disease listed below can be managed, in part, by using passive immunity techniques?
   b.   Hepatitis A infections

5. Mumps viral infections are best controlled in our population by using:
   d.   a live vaccine.

6. Multinucleated giant cells are formed as a result of viral infection. They are formed as a result of viral glycoproteins being added to which host cell structure listed below?
   b.   Cytoplasmic membrane

7. Which viral diseases listed below are currently best controlled by use of vaccines?
   b.   Rubeola and rubella viruses

8. Which respiratory virus listed below can be treated with ribavirin?
   d.   Respiratory syncytial virus

9. A primary viral isolate from a suspected case of poliomyelitis was inoculated into VERO cells, and a dramatic cytopathic effect (CPE) was noted within 24 hours. The isolate was confirmed as poliovirus by neutralization with polyvalent antibody to poliovirus types I, II, III; however, monospecific antibody to each type failed to block CPE. This finding suggests that the isolate contained which of the following?
   d.   Mixture of two types of poliovirus

10. In a serologic test of acute and convalescent sera during a respiratory disease outbreak, the following results were reported. Influenza A—acute <10 and convalescent 10; influenza B—acute <10 and convalescent 40; RSV—acute 10 and convalescent 80. Which conclusion below is correct?
    c.   Two viruses were involved in the outbreak.

CHAPTER 49

Specimen Collection and Processing of Viral Specimens

Suggested Answers to

In a medical center performing organ transplants, patients will often have cytomegalovirus (CMV) reactivation due to immune suppression. If such reactivation occurs, this is important for the managing physician to know because antiviral chemotherapy (ganciclovir) can be given. However, early symptoms of CMV reactivation may be similar to early symptoms of graft rejection, prompting an entirely different patient management regimen to be performed. The patient has recently undergone a liver transplantation and appears to be reacting well to the procedure. One morning, however, he develops an elevated temperature and complains of "not feeling very well." The physician, considering the possibility of CMV infection, orders appropriate specimens to be collected from the patient and sent to the medical center's clinical laboratory for viral studies, including CMV detection. The samples were collected and placed on a bedside deck to be transported to the clinical laboratory. Due to a series of events, the specimens were forgotten for more than 2 days when they were discovered by the nursing staff.

Questions:

1. What specimens are considered appropriate for CMV diagnosis? **Isolation samples would include urine, whole blood (mononuclear cells), and throat swabs. In addition, serum could be collected for serological studies.**

2. Are these specimens still useful as diagnostic material? **Probably not. CMV is considered to be a somewhat fragile virus, which may not survive well in a specimen exposed to even room temperature for several hours. Often** **the number of viruses present in clinical specimens will be relatively few in number.**

3. Under what circumstances would the improperly stored specimens be suitable for valid laboratory diagnostic testing? **If molecular diagnostic techniques (polymerase chain reaction, or PCR) are utilized, the specimens would be suitable for use, since viable viruses are not required.**

Answers to

Review Questions

1. Cytomegalovirus (CMV) is often isolated from whole blood specimens. The part of the specimen that is inoculated onto the human fibroblast cell cultures is:
   b. **mononuclear cells.**

2. Swabs may be used to collect viral isolation samples from all body locations listed below EXCEPT:
   d. **Spinal fluid.**

3. If viral isolation specimens cannot be delivered to a laboratory in a timely manner for processing, what storage condition listed below will be best to maintain viral viability?
   d. **−70°C**

4. Antibiotic pretreatment is usually necessary with some specimens before they can be inoculated into cell cultures. Which specimen listed below MUST be so treated before inoculation?
   d. **Stool**

5. If specimens must be stored in the laboratory before inoculation into cell cultures, what is the maximum length of time they may be kept at 4°C and still be useful diagnostic materials?

   b.   2 days

6. The best temperature used for long-term storage of viruses is:

   d.   −168°C.

7. Toxicity to cell cultures will most likely come from which specimen type listed below?

   c.   Stool specimens

8. Exfoliated cells may be directly examined for viral antigen. Epithelial cells from the respiratory tract are most efficiently collected by which method listed below?

   c.   Biopsy collection

9. Which of the following specimens is not appropriate for general virus isolation?

   a.   Urine

10. Why are swabs with calcium alginate tips not appropriate for the collection of viral specimens?

   b.   Calcium alginate is toxic to herpes simplex viruses.

CHAPTER 50
Clinically Significant Viruses and Their Identification

Suggested Answers to

CASE STUDY

A 9-year-old girl was brought to her pediatrician because of fever and rash for 2 days. She also had a headache, sore throat, coryza, and mild cough. On examination she was alert and in mild distress. Her temperature was 38.3°C, her pulse rate was 110 beats/min, and her respiratory rate was 40/min. She had a mild conjunctivitis. Her posterior pharynx was swollen, and petechiae were present on her soft palate. The buccal mucosa also had scattered raised papular lesions. She had a macular rash on her trunk, face, and arms, and her chest x-ray was normal. A throat culture showed absence of group A streptococci. Acute and convalescent blood samples revealed the diagnosis, and the school nurse was notified.

Questions

1. Which of the following viral infections can present macular rash? Pick all those that apply.
   a. Measles virus
   b. Rubella virus
   c. Roseola virus
   d. EBV
   e. CMV

Answers a, b, and c. Measles (rubeola) and rubella routinely present with a macular rash. Roseola infantum ("sixth disease") also has a similar rash, accompanied by high fever. CMV and EBV do not normally present with a rash.

2. On the basis of the clinical presentation, what is the most likely etiologic agent in this case?
   a. Measles virus
   b. Rubella virus
   c. Roseola virus
   d. EBV
   e. CMV

Answer a, measles (or rubeola) virus is the correct answer.

3. Which of the following information is most significant for you to pick the answer for Question 2?
   a. Fever and rash for 2 days
   b. Headache, sore throat, and mild cough
   c. Throat culture negative for group A streptococci
   d. Coryza, conjunctivitis, and fever

   e. Scattered raised papular lesions on buccal mucosa and palatal petechiae.

Answer e. Many of the symptoms described in the Case Study are general for many viral diseases. The Koplic's spots on the oral buccal and palatal mucosa are specific for measles (rubeola).

4. Currently available methods for preventing this viral infection are:
   a. live attenuated vaccine and passive immunity with pooled human IgG.
   b. killed viral vaccines.
   c. intravenous antiviral drugs.
   d. active and passive immunities with specific toxoids.
   e. nonspecific vaccines to boost cell-mediated immunity.

Answer a. A live-attenuated viral vaccine is available for this disease. Early use of passive immunity is useful if given within 1–3 days after contracting the virus.

5. Which of the following is a *late* complication of this viral infection?
   a. Severe viral encephalitis following rash
   b. Spongiform encephalopathy
   c. Progressive multifocal leukoencephalopathy
   d. Giant cell pneumonia
   e. Subacute sclerosing panencephalitis (SSPE)

Answer e. SSPE has been shown to be caused by a genetic variant of wild type rubeola (measles) virus.

Answers to

Review Questions

1. Reverse transcriptase is involved in the reproduction cycle of which viruses listed below?
   b. HIV and HBV

2. The following serologic tests for hepatitis were reported: HAV IgM positive, HBV$_s$Ag negative, and antibody to HBV$_s$Ag negative. What is your interpretation of the patient's status?
   b. Immune to HAV

3. The most significant respiratory virus for infants less than 6 months old is:
   d. respiratory syncytial virus.

4. Antigenic shift occurs in which virus–antigen combination below?
   d. Mumps virus–fusion protein

5. Killed or inactivated viral vaccines exist for all the following human diseases EXCEPT:
   d. rubella virus.

6. Viruses that can develop a viremia and cross the placenta to infect the fetus include all the following EXCEPT:
   d. respiratory syncytial virus.

7. α-Interferon is approved for use in treating which viral disease listed below?
   b. Hepatitis B

8. Which virus listed below can be accurately described as having a diploid genome?
   d. Human immunodeficiency virus 2

Questions 9 and 10 concern antiviral chemotherapy. Directions: Select the ONE lettered option that is MOST closely associated with the numbered items. Each lettered option may be used once, more than once, or not at all.

   a. Ganciclovir
   b. Acyclovir
   c. Amantadine
   d. Ribavirin
   e. Protease Inhibitors

9. **c. Most effective if used prior to viral entry into the patient.**

10. **b. Effective for varicella-zoster infections**

CHAPTER 51

Emerging Viral Infections

Suggested Answers to

CASE STUDY SEVERE RESPIRATORY ILLNESS

Two weeks after coming home from a camping trip in Arizona, a 21-year-old college student came down with a fever of 102°F and severe muscle aches. She also had a dry cough, headaches, nausea, and vomiting. Four days later the symptoms became progressively worse. Fluid began to accumulate in the lungs. Breathing became more difficult and her blood pressure began to drop. She was then intubated and put on mechanical ventilation.

Serologic and microbiologic tests on various viral and bacterial pathogens were all negative. There was mild thrombocytopenia, leukocytosis, and atypical lymphocytosis. The patient's symptoms were so severe that she had cardiopulmonary arrest and died. Testing of the autopsy specimens were insignificant.

An epidemiologic investigation is conducted. What circumstances should be investigated in regard to her companions, the campsite, and possible related cases?

Questions:

1. What type of investigation of the deceased patient's companions would be appropriate? **Serological tests that screen for antibodies to the Asian hantavirus.**

2. What other investigation should be conducted? **Screen local inhabitants for antibodies to hantavirus.**

3. What would the epidemiologist be looking for at and near the campsite? **Deer mice. They should also investigate the size of the local deer mouse population.**

Answers to

Review Questions

1. Emerging viral infections occur because of:
   d. **All of the above**

2. Which of the following is true?
   c. **The mortality rates of Ebola vary with the subtypes.**

3. Hantavirus pulmonary syndrome:
   b. **is likely a disease that has appeared sporadically throughout the desert southwest, sometimes occurring during years of high rainfall.**

4. Dengue viruses are:
   d. **single-stranded positive-polarity RNA viruses, belonging to the genus *Flavivirus*.**

5. Ebola viruses are:
   a. **enveloped filoviruses with single, negative-stranded RNA.**

6. Hantaviruses are:
   b. **single-stranded RNA viruses that are members of the Bunyaviridae.**

7. The natural reservoir of the Ebola virus is:
   d. **unknown.**

8. Which following statement about dengue is false?

   c. **There is cross-protection between serotypes.**

9. All of the following statements about Hantavirus are true EXCEPT:

   d. **vaccine for Hantavirus is now available.**

10. Infection control measures for Ebola include:

   d. **All of the above.**